AGING
is a
FATAL DISEASE

R C COPELAND

Your body will fight for your health—if you stop sabotaging it. If you're going to live, you may as well make an effort to maintain a healthy body and brain to enjoy the beauty of life. Quality of life has deteriorated for many, however, because of poor health, both physical and mental. Extremism is not necessary—it's not all or nothing—and some reasonable, practical, and inexpensive changes can encourage progress toward ever-better health and substantially delay the processes of aging.

Americans have developed a deadly lifestyle; intentionally ingesting poisons, building new body cells with junk food, and suffering from overweight, underactivity, and diseases of affluence. Americans are seriously malnourished at the same time they are overfed. Joel Fuhrman, M.D. points out that if a program were intentionally developed to destroy health, it would conform almost exactly to American diet and lifestyle. It is making us fat as it slowly kills us.

Section One, **"Here's to Your Good Health!"**, provides a synopsis of a number of good books on nutrition. Good health requires a lifestyle change from the Standard American (SAD) Diet and the intent is to provide as much good information in as brief an analysis as possible. This is a work in progress—there is always more to learn. Even without perfect compliance, you will begin to feel and look so much better!

Section Two, **"The Exercise Advantage"**, provides a simple, short daily program. To feel motivated to do the things you like to do and to have the strength and stamina to do them requires exercise. For those who are motivated, an advanced program, that also takes minimum time and equipment, has been developed.

Section Three, **"Book Outlines"**, provides a number of books related to physical and mental health and relationships. Unfortunately, people struggle more and more in our society to get along effectively with others—and themselves. Body and mind are inextricably linked. A total program for health and youthfulness requires a three-pronged approach, including emotional health as well as nutrition and exercise.

How long do you want to live? How long do you want to live healthy? As well as aging, even advanced states of serious diseases can often be reversed. Are you like Naaman; will you allow ignorance and rationalization to destroy your health? It helps to understand not only *what* to do, but *why*. The best information from twenty good books and many other resources has been condensed into this short book. Nothing worthwhile ever comes easy, but understanding, motivation, commitment, and effort are key. Hopefully, this book will teach you what you need to do and why you need to do it. The commitment and effort are up to you.

TABLE OF CONTENTS

website: tjsbaby.com
© 2011 R C Copeland. vivayo152@yahoo.com

Section One - Here's To YOUR GOOD HEALTH!

AGING *IS* A FATAL DISEASE

Poor health is primarily the result of aging. That conclusion follows from the fact we generally don't have health issues when we are young. The health of a typical American begins at a high point but about age 30 gradually and steadily declines until about age fifty. It then continues at a relatively low level of function, with increasing disease, doctors, and drugs, until a final decline, followed by death, sometime in the seventies. Is that aging model inevitable? Nature intended for health to fall off very slowly, with a relatively high level of function until a rapid drop shortly before death at an advanced age.

The lower line on the following chart illustrates a typical American health plot. The upper line is what nature intended for us. The area between the two lines is the health lost by the typical American who fails to follow principles of good health and nutrition. Which line are you following?

| 0 | 30 | 50 | 70 | 90 |

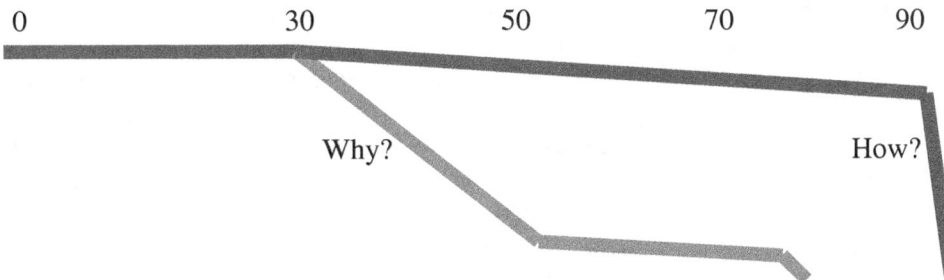

Stephen Cherniske, author of *DHEA Breakthrough*, *Caffeine Blues*, and *The Metabolic Plan*, says health is like a seesaw: When we're young, the repair side is up, the damage side is down and it's easy to be healthy. But the balance starts to tip around age 30, particularly in America, exacerbated by bad diet, excess weight, inactivity, and socially accepted poisons such as caffeine. Thirty-five percent of health is genetic but sixty-five percent is within our control, so our health is our responsibility. Even most genetic issues can be substantially ameliorated.

Americans are slowly digging their grave with their fork and the first thing visitors to America notice is how fat we are. In 1995, no state had an obesity rate above 20%. Now, two-thirds of Americans are overweight and half of those are obese. Most who are not overweight are just fortunate to have "good" genes, as few live an active, nutritionally-healthful lifestyle. Compared to less "advanced" cultures, Americans die primarily from diseases of affluence, including heart disease, cancer, diabetes, and stroke. In one study, 77% of Americans in their *twenties* had signs of incipient heart disease. Young people increasingly are contracting "adult" diseases, such as type-2 diabetes. It doesn't have to happen! In terms of Cherniske's analogy, to remain healthy and youthful we need to find ways to help our bodies press down on the damage side and up on the repair side of the seesaw.

Your body replaces 300 *billion* cells each day, which will be made from whatever you ingest. Aging is the result of cells weakening from damage and poor nutrition and reproducing gradually less healthy cells, as you slowly decay over time. 98% of the cells of your body are replaced each year—what are you rebuilding them with? Obviously, that is a two-edged sword: you can destroy yourself in a year or, to a large extent, begin building a whole new, strong body. You are accountable, in the most direct way, for what you put in your body—you literally are what you eat.

With the exception of a number of great programs on PBS, those who are trusted for advice and support, including the government, health professionals, and public advocates, are often not helpful. Principles that have been accepted, sometimes for generations, turn out to be harmful. We've heard it so long that truth is not even questioned. The source of misinformation, when looked into, is often the food and health industries speaking through a manipulated government. Thomas Jefferson said, "If people let the government decide what foods they eat and what medicines they take, their bodies will soon be in as sorry a state as are the souls who live under tyranny".

Based on recommendations of the government-sponsored National Academy of Science's Food and Nutrition Board—an impressive title— sugar-loaded ketchup was approved as a vegetable and an adequate diet could be, Breakfast: Fruitloops with skim milk, package of peanut M&Ms, and fiber and vitamin supplements. Lunch: Cheeseburger, with ketchup, lettuce, tomato, onions, and pickles, fries, and diet soda. Dinner: Three slices pepperoni pizza, soda, and sugar cookies! Conforming with these recommendations, the average American consumes 62% refined and processed foods and 26% animal and dairy products—and 150 pounds of sugar each year. Investigation by T. Colin Campbell, PhD, for his bestseller *The China Study*, disclosed that 18 of 19 people on the Food and Nutrition Board represented the meat, dairy, and egg industries. They control U.S. government nutrition standards. Similar to how the tobacco industry, for many years, obfuscated the connection between smoking and lung cancer, the Academy labels adverse research "controversial" to confuse the public. Many

2

millions are spent each year by these industries to thwart findings they don't like. Their recommendations are enforced in all Government-financed programs, including school lunches.

Voltaire said, "The art of medicine consists in amusing the patient while nature cures the disease." Doctors and pharmaceutical companies know a lot about disease but very little about health—they are in the "illness industry", treating symptoms and profiting from sickness (Cherniske calls it "symptom stomping"). You've seen the ads on TV, insisting that you, "Ask your doctor if advalorum isn't right for *you!*" They know most doctors can be counted on. One birth control pill has a far higher rate of side effects, including death, than its direct competitor, yet far outsells it. Can you guess why? In 2004, $4 billion was spent on pharmaceutical ads—and more every year—marketing directly to consumers highly complex drugs with serious, esoteric side effects. The head of the National Pharmaceutical Association, at their annual convention, bragged that, "Before the baby boom generation is laid in their graves, they will have spent 50 *trillion* dollars on our products!" He received an enthusiastic standing ovation. The illness industry is approaching *one-fifth* of the total gross national product (GNP). Do you want to add to that statistic?

Chemicals are marketed to alleviate symptoms and doctors are the middlemen. PBS had a program about the one-third of American kids who are overweight. The plan recommended by the National Pediatric Association was to test annually all children older than *two* for cholesterol—and prescribe drugs! Cherniske would ask: "Is high cholesterol a Lipitor deficiency? Is fatigue a caffeine deficiency? Is depression a Prozac deficiency? Is impotence a Viagra deficiency?" Wouldn't it make more sense to look for ways to strengthen our bodies so they are healthy and don't have symptoms that require medical intervention and drugs? On this front of the war, the strategy is not to fight disease but to build a healthy body against which disease cannot establish a beachhead. Dr Timothy Brantley, N.D., PhD maintains, "...disease could not exist or survive in a truly healthy body". According to medical professionals, 70% of heart disease and 80% of cancer could be avoided by good nutrition and health habits. The percentages are probably even higher.

The Nutrition Institute of America published a report showing that in 2001, from the two leading causes, 550,000 Americans died from cancer and 700,000 died from heart disease. Almost 800,000 died from medical treatment, including misdiagnoses, botched medical procedures, and reactions to drugs. Medical malpractice is actually the leading cause of death in America. In addition, over 2.2 million were injured by improperly prescribed drugs and their side effects. Acetaminophen, for example, is the leading cause of liver failure, at 56,000 per year. As someone sarcastically said, we should ban doctors, not guns—and the predatory pharmaceutical companies. But once bad health habits bring on the symptoms of disease, they've got you.

Nutrition is a complex and controversial subject, with a new fad nearly every week. For example, there is a recent study that "proves" caffeine is good for you and the more coffee you drink, the better. Responsible parents, even though they drink it, will not allow their children to drink coffee, knowing it is not good for them but, according to this study, coffee is even good for young children. Very persuasive—until you find that the study was funded by the coffee industry. Responsible mothers really want the very best for their families, but in a sea of misinformation, controversy, and greed it is almost impossible. It is tempting, and certainly easier, simply to give up and go along. But it is too important—you are literally betting your life, as well as your ability to function effectively and without pain. The world is full of experts; how is one to know whom to listen to? By studying numerous authorities, looking for consensus, questioning motives, examining qualifications, and applying some common sense (which Will Rogers quipped is not too common) reasonable conclusions can be reached and then tested. That is the approach of this book: to find universal elements for establishing and maintaining good health and youthfulness. Ten really good books and hundreds of articles have been thoroughly studied. Some of the information is no doubt incorrect—this is such a complex and controversial subject—but the overall program undoubtedly provides the best program for good health and it dovetails with the Word of Wisdom.

People often like to think they are unique—that tests and diagnoses are required to prescribe for their individual issues. Certainly, if there are serious symptoms or genetic propensities, medical diagnosis may be critical. Tests can show specific supplements to take, by analyzing levels of hormones, enzymes, vitamins, and minerals to determine deficiencies. Testing, however, is expensive. A SPECT brain scan, for example, costs $3000 and dozens of other possible tests cost up to $200 each or more. That approach is much like the medical industry practice of treating symptoms rather than creating healthy bodies that do not need drugs. Dr Roger Williams, distinguished as a researcher who discovered some of the vitamins, found that requirements for various nutrients can vary among individuals by as much as 40 times. One person may require 2.5mg of V-B5, for example, while another requires 100mg. "Recommended levels" are therefore meaningless. It is also argued that RDA levels have been set very low by the FDA in order to make the essentially nutritionless food of a SAD diet appear better than it is. The results experienced by those who take highly concentrated fruits and vegetables prove that huge concentrations of nutritious natural foods (not supplements) can have amazing health results.

There is an ad that says, "You can pay me now, or pay me later!" The price to be paid later for poor health habits is frightening, and early death is not the worst of it—many older Americans are experiencing years of living death. Of course, the price to be paid now for good health is not particularly easy either, but it is generally the same for everyone: Eat nutrient-rich foods, give up or substantially reduce your favorite toxins and addictions, like sugar, refined food, soda, meat, and dairy products, take a few appropriate supplements, and exercise. Does that seem too restrictive and difficult? You may agree with the old joke of the man bragging about his healthy lifestyle: Early to bed and early to rise, ate only the plainest foods, drank only water, walked five miles every day, no bad habits, avoided all risk—he intended to live to be a hundred. "Why would you want to?", someone pointedly asked. Your choice. Do you prefer obesity, pain, disease, drugs, surgery, and early death? Is there a reasonable compromise?

To keep it as simple as possible, a few basic things can get you on the road to good nutritional health. (A short-list is provided in the section "The Bottom Line".) As health begins to improve, motivation, understanding, and compliance gradually increase. To start, it is not too difficult to shop for healthy food, substituting whole grains, whole-wheat pasta, and brown rice instead of their refined varieties, to eat more fresh fruits and vegetables instead of sugar, junk food, and processed foods, to drink plenty of lemon water instead of soda, and to take a few basic supplements. Don't jump into it, grow into it.

It is never too early or too late to start, but the older you get the more important it becomes. You don't need to be perfect to succeed and once you start feeling better and your health improves you will be encouraged to continue. Rationalization is one of the greatest human skills, but knowledge is power and the more you learn, the better judgments you can make and the more you will be motivated to make them. It has been proven that those who take a proactive role in researching and determining treatments for their own health, even for esoteric ailments, are most likely to be healthy and to recover from disease. You need to look for support from the growing "wellness industry" to build a healthy body, rather than rely on the "illness industry" to treat symptoms. Hopefully this book will provide a foundation from which to develop and follow your own plan. In serious cases, certainly, this needs to be done in consultation with a medical expert.

THE AGING SEESAW

Cherniske's "seesaw" of health describes two opposing facets: damage and repair. Our bodies, working at the cellular level, are constantly metabolizing the food we eat. Simplistically, metabolism takes two forms: anabolic and catabolic. Anabolic metabolism, which prevails in youth, builds and repairs the body, generates energy, and fights aging and disease. Catabolic metabolism, after about age thirty or so, becomes more and more dominant. It damages cells, and even DNA, resulting in reproduction of defective cells and aging. Looking at the damage side of the seesaw, there are four causes; each is insidious and cumulates as we become older. To counteract these, the repair side is increasingly necessary, through a nutritious diet and avoidance of toxins.

Oxidation. Oxidants in cells, called "free radicals", result from all normal metabolic functions but, when out of control, they are also involved in all diseases. They are atoms or molecules with an unpaired electron seeking attachment, which results in damage to healthy molecules, even including DNA. An oxidative chain reaction is begun, as more and more healthy molecules are affected, and the body becomes less healthy and ages. Good nutrition provides sufficient antioxidants, with donor electrons, to counteract normal metabolic processes, but poor nutrition and toxins destroy the balance. The worst oxidants, in approximately descending order, are alcohol, nicotine, caffeine, refined sugar, saturated fats, animal products, processed foods, refined grains, and pharmaceutical drugs. It is essentially impossible for the body to provide enough antioxidants to counteract the cumulation of these, so they need to be avoided. The Government has devised the "ORAC Score" (Oxygen Radical Absorbance Capacity) to test antioxidants and lists are available online to determine which foods are best. There is great variability, but the best anti-oxidants are found in fruits and vegetables, particularly spices, and Vitamin-A, V-C, and V-E. One of the better ones, better than vaunted blueberries, is chocolate. Just eat it without sugar! The highest anti-oxidant is cloves, followed by cinnamon, oregano, and turmeric.

Inflammation. Time magazine had a cover story calling inflammation "The Silent Killer", and its terrible effects are beginning to be recognized. It is the body's defense against disease, attacking invaders and damaged body cells, but it becomes over-aggressive, attacking healthy cells as well. This is particularly so when the attacked cells are similar to the body's own cells, such as meat and dairy products. Inflammation damages organs, muscles and joints, and is a companion of most diseases, increasing their effects. It is the mechanism by which cancer spreads. It inhibits nutrients, even when they are available, from getting into damaged cells to nourish them (a reason glucosamine does not work for some people.) In autoimmune diseases, the body triggers inflammation that attacks its own tissues indiscriminately. Body fat as well as injuries and infection produce inflammation, and many foods are inflammatory, particularly animal protein, saturated fats, refined grains, sugar, and toxins such as tobacco, caffeine and alcohol. Again, the best natural anti-inflammatories are fruits and vegetables, such as sorghum bran, broccoli and decaf green tea. Among the highest are turmeric, ginger, and olive oil.

Infection. When our bodies do not have the nutrients or cellular energy to maintain natural defenses, inflammation and oxidation promote infection. Infection increases as the immune system declines from age, toxins, and a SAD diet. Poor dental hygiene is a serious, but often unsuspected, cause of infection, and many diseases throughout the body, including cardio-vascular disease, cancer, and autoimmune diseases, are exacerbated by it. Refined sugar drastically reduces white blood cell count in the bloodstream and healthful bacteria in the GI tract, which is the body's first line of defense. Antibiotics have been developed to defend against bacteria, but they are not effective against viruses, and medical science has no real answer to them. Natural antibodies, not drugs, should be the body's primary defense to all pathogens, and a healthy body develops its own natural systems to fight infection and disease, including both bacteria and viruses. Though many exaggerated claims have been made, a combination of cinnamon and unpasteurized honey, taken daily, fights infections and fungus. Cranberry juice, cayenne pepper, and probiotic supplements are also effective.

Stress. We experience two types of stress: Stress from living and stress on our cells and organs. Stress from life is unavoidable in our world and is highly damaging, as it reduces energy, contributes to an acidic imbalance, and weakens the immune system, promoting inflammation and infection. Toxins, bacteria, viruses, and stimulants increase stress at the cellular level. Coffee, caffeinated sodas, and "energy" drinks provide a body-damaging short-term energy lift. A recent study shows the combination of caffeine and stress can cause symptoms of psychosis. Just observe activity on our highways. It is important to develop ways to de-stress, including adequate sleep, deep breathing, meditation, self-discipline, exercise, and laughter (which can also reduce inflammation).

GENETICS VS. DIET

At any given age, some people look younger and are obviously healthier than others. Although genes are implicated, they do not usually cause disease and early aging, they just predispose them. People with "good genes" can often abuse their bodies for years with little apparent affect, but it is Russian roulette. Increasingly with age, genetic "triggers" like poor nutrition, toxins, and other illnesses often determine whether diseases are activated. They are the key to controlling the 35% of health that is genetic. For example, as documented by *The China Study*, animal proteins in the bloodstream, from foods, are often the trigger. Our bodies build antibodies to attack them—and then begin attacking the body itself, since the proteins are similar.

Good diet is our single most powerful weapon for good health, even against genetically predisposed illnesses. Reducing animal protein is critical to live longer and healthier, arrest and reverse disease, look younger, have more energy, lose weight, increase mental acuity—and avoid drugs and doctors. It is ironic that the wealthiest nation on earth has some of the deadliest foods. It is very difficult in our society to follow good nutrition practices, but the better they are followed the greater will be the positive effect on health. *The China*

Study determined that, even with genetic predisposition:

- People who eat the least animal products and the most unprocessed plant foods get the least disease.
- Conversely, people who eat the most animal products get the most disease. This is exacerbated by all the growth hormones, antibiotics, and other chemicals fed to animals.
- The same diet, including food and supplements, that is good for avoiding one disease is generally good for all others.
- Heart disease, diabetes, cancer, autoimmune diseases, etc. can often be substantially *reversed* with proper diet.
- Dairy products, particularly cow's milk when young or genetically predisposed, greatly increase risk of disease, including diabetes for children. [A recent study, however, indicates that feeding soy-based formula to male infants encourages permanent brain changes toward those of girls, so that may not be a good option. Obviously, mother's milk, for as long as possible, is best.]
- Even after a month on a primarily plant-based diet, you will be healthier, look better, feel better, and begin to lose weight.

A study of eighteen people who had suffered, collectively, 49 serious coronary events put them on a plant-based diet, with no drugs. After eleven years there was only one subsequent event, an angina attack, from a patient who stopped following the diet.

Type-2 diabetes used to be called "adult onset", but it is occurring in younger and younger people. The pancreas stops producing insulin, often influenced by obesity. Diet is crucial to diabetics, particularly reducing animal proteins and sugar and increasing whole, unrefined plant food. Deaths from diabetes are reduced by this diet from 20.4/100,000 to 2.9/100,000. After only three weeks, type-1 diabetics lowered insulin medication up to 40%, and most type-2 diabetics stopped insulin entirely (24 of 25 in one study).

Cancer studies show much higher incidence in societies eating more animal protein and Americans average over 200 pounds of meat per year. Many chemicals are carcinogens, but cancer often is triggered by animal proteins in the bloodstream. In lab tests, for example, rats were fed aflatoxin, a cancer-causing chemical. Of those receiving 20% animal protein in their diet, from cow's milk, *all* got cancer; of those receiving only 5% animal protein, *none* did. (More than 20% animal protein is what Americans consume as a typical diet, and our Government recommends up to 35%! Remember who controls Government standards? An old story is told of a farmer who liked steak even for breakfast, commenting that, "You need plenty of meat to build strong muscles and bones". He then harnessed up his mules to plow his field…)

In the aflotoxin test, cancer could even be turned on and off in the rats, like a switch, by feeding or withholding animal protein. All forms of cancer were subject to the same effects of diet, both pro and con. Breast cancer, for example, has been linked to high levels of female hormones, and eating animal protein increases these. It has also been noted that cancer increases with distance from the equator. A recent British study showed vitamin D, from the sun or supplements, can arrest, and even reverse, cancer. Virtually all Americans are deficient.

Autoimmune diseases, including hyper/hypo-thyroid, MS, arthritis, lupus, type-1 diabetes, Crohn's disease, etc., are genetically predisposed and are newly diagnosed in 250,000 Americans each year. The body attacks itself, often triggered by a virus. These diseases are also more prevalent farther from the equator, with less V-D, and with increased use of animal protein, including cow's milk. If caught in early stages, they can be reversed; and slowed if caught later. With proper diet and lifestyle before the onset of symptoms of these and other diseases, it can be expected that the symptoms will not occur, even with genetic predisposition.

MACRONUTRIENTS

Nutrients include macronutrients—protein, carbohydrates, and fats—and micronutrients, contained in macronutrients—vitamins, minerals, and phytochemicals. Good nutrients, including micronutrients, are necessary for energy, to build healthy new cells, and to develop immunity from disease. A good diet plans for adequate amounts of each, and supplements are available for many of these when diet is not sufficient to provide them and as aging reduces metabolism. Though many try to maintain a Standard American (SAD) Diet and counteract it with supplements, a proper diet is superior to most supplements, and many micronutrients can be obtained only from food. Good nutrition is almost always superior to drugs and supplements.

Macronutrients are the primary constituents of diet. They include protein, carbohydrates, and fats and are the source of all calories. When properly digested, proteins are broken down into amino acids, carbohydrates into glucose, and fats into glycerin and fatty acids.

Proteins are obtained from both animals and plants. They provide fuel as well as material for the body to build and repair itself. There are ten "non-essential" amino acids, meaning that the body can synthesize them from other nutrients, and ten "essential" amino acids that must be obtained directly from food. Animal proteins are "complete" in that they provide all the essential amino acids; plant proteins, with the exception of soy, often must be obtained from numerous types of plants to obtain all essential amino acids. On the other hand, animal protein has no fiber, is high in unhealthy saturated fats, and, in modern society, is loaded with toxins. Eating meat creates an acid

9

condition in the body, ideal for growth of cancer and other diseases. It also substantially increases the rate of aging. Processed meats are particularly toxic.

Besides other issues involving animal protein, American meat, beef, pork, poultry, milk, and eggs are loaded with growth hormones. Why do you suppose American children reach puberty earlier and earlier? Early puberty, together with animal products in the bloodstream, has been shown to correlate with breast, prostate, testicular cancers and early death. Most meat is also loaded with antibiotics and toxins. Seafood is not necessarily much of an improvement. Farm-raised fish has the same "additives" as meat and is highly oxidative, and native fish often has mercury or other toxins. People who eat a lot of meat, including fish and poultry, are twice as likely to develop dementia.

It is best to obtain most protein from plant sources and reduce quantities of meat and other animal proteins, including milk and, particularly, cheese. Ten percent animal protein in the diet seems to be the maximum without incurring bad health effects. Textured vegetable protein (TVP) soaked in bouillon can be substituted in recipes requiring ground beef. Used in spaghetti sauce or nachos, it is indistinguishable from ground beef.

Carbohydrates are either "simple" or "complex" and are metabolized into sugar for fuel. Simple carbohydrates include refined sugar and refined grains. These contain little or no fiber or micronutrients and require little energy for the body to turn into glucose. They provide little nutrition, except calories, suppress the immune system, and overwork the pancreas. As a major component of diet, they may lead to fatigue, obesity, diabetes, oral diseases, heart disease, and other ailments. They are oxidative, inflammatory, and encourage infection. Honey and fruits are also relatively simple sugars but, as well as providing micronutrients, antioxidants, anti-microbials, and other health benefits, they provide a more stable blood sugar level than other simple sugars. Honey is approximately equal in fructose and sucrose, allowing the liver to store it as glycogen and slowly release it for energy.

Complex carbohydrates require an energy-burning process to digest and convert to simple sugars. This leads to a fuller feeling when eating, which is good for those on a diet, and a more stable blood sugar balance. Complex carbohydrates have many more nutrients, including vitamins and minerals, than simple carbohydrates, animal proteins, or fats, and also contain phytonutrients, such as flavenoids and chlorophyll. These are powerful anti-oxidants and some can metabolize toxins, allowing them to be excreted. Others help prevent many diseases, including cancer, cardiovascular disease, etc. The fiber in complex carbohydrates is necessary for proper digestive and excretory processes, and fiber helps bind fat and toxins in the body for excretion. Non-soluble fiber accomplishes this in the intestine and soluble fiber performs a similar task in the vascular system where it also helps reduce cholesterol.

A healthful diet should include a wide variety of 1) whole grains, such as whole wheat ("wheat" bread is not whole wheat), instead of refined grains, 2) brown rice instead of white, 3) whole-wheat pasta, 4) beans and other legumes, 5) many different fruits and vegetables, all of which have different combinations of nutrients. Plant food must be washed carefully, as America uses a billion pounds of pesticides each year, which can cause serious disease. Food should not be over-cooked or cooked in excess water, as it destroys nutrients.

Fats are required in much lesser amounts than proteins or carbohydrates, but are necessary for energy and cell metabolism. They are essential for the brain, eyes, vascular system, nerve system, kidneys, hair, skin, nails, mood, hormone synthesis, anti-inflammation, and immunity. An Australian study demonstrated that eating polyunsaturated fats reduced symptoms of ADHD in 132 children, including inattention, hyperactivity, and impulsivity.

There are three types of fats: monounsaturated fats, such as olive oil and peanut oil, polyunsaturated fats, such as oil from fish, flax, and soy, and saturated fats, the bad ones, such as oil from meat, butter, and margarine. The first two types are necessary for good health, but saturated fat, which is a solid or semi-solid at room temperature, can lead to cancer, cardiovascular disease, stroke, inflammation, and a plethora of other diseases. Body fat is also a storage medium for toxins in the body.

There are three groups of fatty acids necessary for health: Omega 3, Omega 6, and Omega 9. O-3 is the most important for health and the best source is fish oil and fatty fish, such as salmon. There are many sources of O-6, and a SAD diet is backward as it provides 10-30 times as much of this as O-3. Excess levels contribute to all the same diseases attributed to saturated fat. O-9 is provided by olive and canola oils, but can be synthesized by the body, so it is not required to be directly ingested.

There are a total of twenty acids among O-3, O-6, and O-9. The body can synthesize all but two of these from nutrients provided by a good diet. It can only minimally synthesize DHA, which is the most important. ALA (alphalinolenic acid) and LA (linoleic acid) must be obtained directly from foods containing them. ALA can be obtained from fish (which also provides DHA) and flaxseed oil and LA can be obtained from safflower and corn oils. Canola (rapeseed) oil has both. Toxins, sugar, and refined grains deplete these nutrients. Deficiency can encourage arthritis, asthma, A.D.D., cardiovascular disease, stroke, cancer, depression, skin disorders, diabetes, fatigue, baldness, hypertension, memory loss, and schizophrenia.

Good nutrition involves adequate amounts of healthful forms of each of the three macronutrients, emphasizing those that are nutrient-rich and contain substantial micronutrients. A change of lifestyle is usually required, as it is a total contradiction of the SAD diet to which Americans are literally addicted, but once the habit is established it is not particularly difficult. Perfection is not required, but the better you do, the better you will feel and the healthier you will be. Prove it! Try it consistently for just one month, or even follow Dr Fuhrman's six-week program, in the section on weight loss, and see how much better you feel. This diet can be less expensive than a SAD diet, provided food is bought in quantity and not from health-food stores. Only healthful foods should be purchased, avoiding the temptation of having unhealthful versions in the house. Read labels and avoid refined grains, sugar, preservatives, and saturated or hydrogenated oils. Care should be taken in selection and preparation of all foods, and argument can certainly be made for organically grown food.

Water is not considered a macronutrient, but it would seem it should be. You are not just what you eat; you are what you drink, and water is the primary constituent of the body. Muscles and brain, for example, are 75% water and blood is 82% water. Even mild dehydration causes fatigue and three-fourths of Americans are chronically dehydrated. Thirst is often mistaken for hunger. If you wait till you are thirsty to drink water, you are already dehydrated.

Many diseases can be caused or exacerbated by dehydration and can therefore be prevented or treated by increasing water intake. Some of these may seem surprising. Possible examples include: Fatigue, heartburn, ulcers, arthritis, lower back pain, joint pain, muscle cramps, angina, migraines, constipation, colitis, hemorrhoids, asthma, high blood pressure, type-2 diabetes, and high cholesterol. Often, drugs treat symptoms that could be treated simply—and better—just by drinking more water. Even if they alleviate the condition, drugs may cause other long-term injury to the body from resulting inflammation, oxidation, infection, and stress.

The usual recommendation is eight glasses (64 ounces) a day, more for larger people, and ½ ounce for each pound of body weight in the event of high activity and heat. (In extreme conditions, the body can sweat a quart an hour and if sweating stops, death is imminent.) A recent survey claimed Americans average $2500 per year on bottled water. Ridiculous! Bottled water comes from municipal systems and may or may not be pure. A test of 100 brands showed a large percentage contained minute quantities of toxins and bacteria. Tap water can easily be filtered, and sitting in an open container in the refrigerator also allows chlorine, which is a major contaminant in most tap water, to escape. This is important as, among other things, chlorine kills the good bacteria in the gastro-intestinal system. Many do not like to drink water and take soda, coffee, or tea instead. Along with other bad effects, these actually dehydrate the body and contribute to acidity. A recent study shows diet drinks actually *increase* the level of sugar in the bloodstream and lead to weight gain. Add lemon or lime juice to water—no sugar—for healthful flavoring.

Fiber, the indigestible component of plants, is also not considered a nutrient, but large amounts are essential for health. Almost everyone is deficient in fiber and it is critical to immunity as well as elimination of waste and toxins. Constipation results from insufficient fiber and this can be a chronic problem resulting in a steady buildup of toxins in the large intestine and in other parts of the body. Many diseases are directly or indirectly attributable to lack of sufficient fiber in the diet. Cultures that have a high fiber intake—from high-fiber *foods*, not supplements—have virtually none of the diseases of affluent societies, including heart disease and cancer.

There are two types of fiber: soluble (in water) and insoluble. Both are important and eating a variety of fruits and vegetables is the best way to obtain them. Dr Fuhrman recommends a minimum of 50 grams a day, from foodits. Soluble fiber is absorbed into the bloodstream and acts as a kind of sponge, absorbing toxins. As it passes through the system, it regulates the absorption of sugar and it reduces cholesterol. Insoluble fiber, "roughage", moves bulk through the intestinal tract and helps balance pH.

pH balance has caused a good deal of discussion and concern recently. Proper balance is best achieved through macronutrients, and test strips for saliva and urine are available to check it. Ph ranges in nature between 0, acid, and 14, alkaline. A slightly alkaline body, about 7.2 to 7.4, is optimum, though there are daily variations, with early morning often being just slightly acidic. The maximum range for urine is 4.5 – 8.5. Many diseases and undesirable conditions may result from the acidic, anaerobic condition that is created by a SAD diet: It interferes with metabolism, including cell nutrition, energy, and healthy cell growth. It encourages propagation of bacteria, viruses, fungus, and mold. Cancer thrives. The body may grow fat cells in self-defense to the acid environment, as fat stores acid. Osteoporosis is often caused by an acidic body, as the body robs calcium from bones to maintain a survivable pH level. Calcium deposits, paradoxically, are not the result of too much calcium, but too little.

A diet of approximately 20% acid and 80% alkaline is considered best, and the SAD diet is backward. Meat, dairy, sugar, and grain form acids; vegetables and fruits (even citrus, such as water with a shot of lemon) form alkalines. A substantially plant-based diet, without any other intervention, will achieve an ideal pH balance.

Food Allergies and Sensitivities are toxic reactions to food or food additives and are estimated to be involved in up to half of difficult-to-diagnose chronic symptoms. They can cause virtually any symptom in any part of the body and should be suspected in the event of any chronic condition. They may be caused by an inappropriate or over-active response of the immune system or by lack of a digestive enzyme. Llactose intolerance, for example, prevents milk from being digested. Frank Oski, M.D., former head of Pediatrics at Johns Hopkins, in his book *Don't Drink Your Milk*, claims that dairy products are a major cause of food sensitivities and are always the cause of, for example, continuing strep throat. There is a substantial list of foods causing sensitivities, but dairy, wheat, and peanuts are probably the most common.

There are several tests for determining food allergies, but none is entirely certain. A self-test can be made by an elimination diet of eating only non-allergenic food and then adding foods back in one at a time. Foods that are nearly always safe include lamb, fish (not shellfish), rice, potatoes, buckwheat, all vegetables except corn, and all fruits except citrus. After five to ten days, each day eat a large portion of the questioned food at every meal and observe any symptoms. If joint pain is a symptom, add a new food every two days. Very occasionally, symptoms may take as long as five days to occur.

Gluten is a popular food allergy these days. It is a protein in wheat, rye, and barley that is recognized by chewiness and elasticity in the dough. When a person with an autoimmune condition known as "celiac disease" eats gluten, the lining of the small intestine becomes inflamed and damaged. Absorption of nutrients is reduced, which can lead to malnutrition, osteoporosis, tooth decay, weight loss, and other serious issues. Lesser problems, which can indicate presence of the disease or of gluten sensitivity, include diarrhea, stomach upset, abdominal pain, and bloating. It is estimated that one of every 130 people is sensitive to gluten, though symptoms for most people are minor. The disease may take years to diagnose because doctors mistake it for irritable bowel syndrome or other diseases and lab tests are often inconclusive. Since the subject has become a fad, some insist a gluten-free diet is healthier, but that is not the case for people who do not have a sensitivity. A gluten-free diet is difficult to follow and may cause nutritional deficiencies for people with no medical reason to be on it. If symptoms indicate possible gluten sensitivity, avoid products containing them for a few weeks and observe whether there is an improvement.

MICRONUTRIENTS

Micronutrients, which basically include vitamins, minerals, and phytochemicals, are critically important for health. Vegetables, fruits, whole grains, herbs, and spices are the primary source of these, though supplements can provide vitamins and minerals. Amounts in natural sources vary, but many plant products provide 100 times more of these important nutrients than the best animal products and many can be obtained only from plants. They are imperative in fighting disease and, incidentally, many inhibit excessive growth of fat cells.

Vitamins are organic substances essential for life. Most cannot be synthesized by the body and must be obtained from food or supplements. Fat-soluble vitamins, A, D, K, and E, are stored longer than water-soluble vitamins, which are easily excreted and must be replenished regularly. It is possible to overdose with supplements of some fat-soluble vitamins.

Vitamin	Typical Dose	Function	Natural Source	Toxic if O.D?
A	2-5000iu	Vision, growth, immunity	Vegetables: Betacarotene	Y! @ 25,000 iu
B1 Thiamin	5-10 mg	Energy, nerves, brain, heart	Grains, meat, legumes	N
B2 Riboflavin	10-15 mg	Energy, metabolism	Organs, fish, whole grain, vegetables	N
B3 Niacin (Niacinamide is best)	50-100 mg,	Energy, blood, mood, cognition, arthritis	Organs, fish, grain, peanuts, poultry	Y @ 2000iu
B5	50-100 mg	Metabolism, adrenal hormones, blood	Organs, fish, chicken, grains, vegetables	N
B6	10-25 mg	Proteins, nerves, blood, immunity	Grains, soy, poultry, potatoes	Min. @ 400mg
B9 Folic Acid	400-800 mcg	DNA, Metabolism, energy, cardiovascular, blood, skin, nails, anti-cancer, men's fertility	Leafy vegetables	N
B12	50-200 mcg	DNA, blood, nerves	Seafood, soy, synthesized in digestion	N
Biotin	300 mcg	Metabolism, nails, hair	Organs, wheat peanuts	N
C (Ascorbic acid)	500-1500 mg	Antioxident, immunity, collagen, bones, anti-cancer, etc.	Citrus, potatoes, etc	Diarrhea
CoQ10*	30-200 mg	95% of energy, antioxidant, cardio-vascular, etc.	Fish, organs, oils, nuts, fruit	Y @ >3600mg
D [D3 is	400-800	Bones, immunity,	Sunlight,	Y @

15

best]	iu	thyroid	fish, fish oil	4000 IU
E	400 iu	Antioxident, immunity, blood, nerves	Oils, seeds, nuts, brn. rice, grains	N
K	50-100 mcg	Antioxident, blood, bones	Vegetables, soy, legumes, synthesized in digestion	Y
Carotenoids (600)	5-25000 iu	Antioxident, immunity, V-A, tissue growth	Vegetables, fruits	N

*The FDA decided all vitamins had been found, so they could not recognize CoQ10 as one.

Minerals are inorganic substances that affect vitamins, hormones, enzymes, and metabolism. They are 4 percent of body weight and a particularly important constituent in bones. Sea salt is a good source.

Mineral	Typical Dose	Function	Natural Source	Toxic if O.D?
Calcium	1000-1500 mg	Bones, teeth, nerves, muscles, heart, blood	Kelp, vegetables, soy, almonds	N
Choline	500 mg	Nerves, metabolism	Liver, chicken, caulifower	Min.
Chromium	200 mcg	Blood sugar, energy	Grains, meat, potatoes	N
Copper	2-3 mg	Collagen, blood, bones, energy, brain, etc.	Grains, organs, shellfish, poultry, legumes	Min.
Iodine	250 mcg	Thyroid	Seafood, iodized salt	Y
Iron	1-20 mg	Blood, collagen, immunity	Organs, beef, legumes	Y
Magnesium	400-600 mg	Bones, teeth, energy, muscles, nerves, metabolism	Grains, nuts, legumes, soy	N?
Manganese	5-10 mg	Energy, blood sugar, metabolism, thyroid, bones, tissue repair	Organs, grains, vegetables	Y
Molybdenum	200	Metabolism	Meat, grains	N

	mcg			
Phosphorus	800-1200 mg	Growth, bones, energy, kidneys	Meat, fish, eggs, poultry	Min.
Potassium	2-3000 mg	Nerves, pH, heart, kidneys, adrenal glands	Fruits, vegetables, potatoes, meat, fish	Y
Selenium	200 mcg	Antioxidant, anti-cancer, immunity, thyroid	Seafood, grains, organs, vegetables	Y
Silicon	50 mg	Bones, cartilage, ligaments, skin	Grains, roots	N
Sodium	2000 mg	pH, muscles, nerves, amino acid absorption	Ubiquitous	Min.
Vanadium	50 mg	Blood sugar, bones, teeth	Shellfish, pepper	N?
Zinc	15-30 mg	Enzyme reactions, hormones, immunity, healing, metabolism, vision	Seafood, meat, grains, legumes, nuts	Min.

Phytochemicals, also called phytonutrients, are produced, as the name says, *only* in plants. Ten thousand have been identified and there are more. Flavonoids, for example, are phytochemicals that give flowers and fruits their vibrant colors and protect them from microbial and insect attack. Consumption of foods containing phytochemicals has been linked to many health benefits. They remove toxins from cells and help the body protect itself from virtually all diseases. Though they provide minimal antioxident benefit, due to slow absorption by the body, they trigger the production of natural enzymes that fight disease, including flu, tooth decay, cancer, heart disease, and age-related degenerative diseases. Phytochemicals are generally not available in supplements and can only be obtained by eating a wide variety of fruits and vegetables of many colors. Kale tops the list. Excess cooking destroys them, so it is best to eat many plant foods raw (except tomatoes have better lycopene if cooked). Dr Fuhrman, another advocate for acronyms as a memory device, says the best foods for phytochemicals and disease protection spell "GOMBS": Greens, Onions, Mushrooms, Beans/Berries, and Seeds.

PLANT FOODS

Fruits and Vegetables are the best sources of nutrition. As well as macronutrients, all fruits and vegetables, in varying amounts, are anti-inflammatory, anti-oxidant, and contain micronutrients that boost metabolism and the immune system. Almost all contain soluble or insoluble fiber. Be sure foods are carefully cleaned and not overcooked. Eat them raw whenever possible or steam rather than boil. It is important to eat lots of different varieties and colors. You may even want to grow a small garden, for the freshest healthful and inexpensive foods. Pigments tell a story:

Red fruits and vegetables contain lycopene, ellagic acid, quercetin, and hesperidin. They reduce blood pressure, tumor growth, cholesterol, and risk of prostate cancer and arthritis.

Orange and yellow fruits and vegetables contain beta-carotene, zeaxanthin, lycopene, potassium, and V-C. They protect from macular degeneration, prostate cancer, cholesterol, and high blood pressure. They promote collagen, healthy joints, alkaline balance, and, with magnesium and calcium, build healthy bones.

Green fruits and vegetables (usually the darker the better) contain chlorophyll, fiber, lutein, zeaxanthin, folate, V-C, calcium, beta-carotene, and calcium. They clean out cells, aid healing, and reduce cancer risk, blood pressure, and cholesterol. They assist bone health, digestion, vision, and immunity.

Blue and purple fruits and vegetables contain anthocyanin, lutein, zeaxanthin, resveratrol, ellagic acid, and quercetin. They reduce cholesterol, tumor growth, and cancer risk in the GI tract. They support vision, immunity, digestion, and mineral absorption.

It is very difficult to make a list of "best" fruits and vegetables, but here are some that are generally available and favored:

Fruits: 1. Apples 2. Raisins 3. Berries 4. Kiwi 5. Bananas 6. Melons 7. Plums 8. Oranges 9. Red grapes 10. Cherries.

Vegetables: 1. Kale 2. Onions 3. Brussel sprouts 4. Asparagus 5. Broccoli 6. Beets 7. Red bell peppers 8. Spinach 9. Avocados 10. Eggplant.

Spices and Herbs contain some of the highest concentrations of micronutrients, including phytochemicals. A German proverb says a garden is the poor man's apothecary, so use lots of them to season food. They also help kill any bacteria in food. Some are available as supplements or you can buy empty capsules and make your own.

Spices:
Basil: Antioxidant, vitamin A, iron, calcium, vitamin C, and magnesium. Helps healthy blood flow.
Cayenne: Circulation, infection. Available as an analgesic cream.
Cilantro: Goes by several names, including coriander. Can be eaten from root to tip. Sprinkle the leaves into salsas or curries and use the seeds to add a warm, citrus flavor to foods. Regulates blood sugar and cholesterol, is antibacterial, and aids in detox of heavy metals.

Cinnamon (especially with unpasteurized honey): High anti-oxidant, helps defend cardio-vascular disease, cholesterol, arthritis, bladder infection, colds and flu, upset stomach, immune system, weight loss, and hearing loss.

Garlic: Anti-viral, anti-fungal, anti-bacterial, fights cholesterol, ear infection, and heart disease.

Ginger: Anti-inflammatory, anti-oxidant, and anti-nausea.

Mint: Sore throats, congestion, itching, and minor aches and pains. The oil of peppermint soothes stomach upset by calming muscle spasms, such as IBS.

Oregano: Antioxidant, iron, calcium, omega-3 fatty acids, and vitamin K.

Parsley: Anti-oxidant, folic acid, V-A, and V-C.

Rosemary: Antioxidant. Excellent for skin and protects against UV-A. May protect from stroke, Alzheimer's, and other age-related degenerative conditions.

Sage: Boosts brain power. Its oil enhanced research participants' instant recall and compounds in its roots may help to inhibit the growth of brain plaques that form in Alzheimer's.

Thyme: Antioxidant. May support healthy brain function by boosting omega-3 fatty acids in brain.

Turmeric: Common to all curry powders. The distinctive yellow pigment, curcumin, has been recognized for its excellent anti-inflammatory, antioxidant, and anti-infection properties. It provides tumor inhibition, enhances liver function, Strengthens cell immunity and DNA, aids detoxification, reduces pain, inhibits stomach ulcers, and fights cancer. It inhibits the oxidative damage that leads to Parkinson's disease, can counteract DNA damage caused by arsenic, may help protect against type 2 diabetes and reduce the dangerous inflammation associated with obesity and reduce the chance of developing heart failure as well as preventing and reversing hypertrophy (enlarged heart).

Herbs:

Alfalfa: Arthritis, cholesterol, anemia, skin disorders.

Aloe Vera: External for burns and wounds; internal for digestive disorders, diabetes.

Ashwaganda: Full of flavenoids. Strong anti-oxidant, anti-inflammatory. Strengthens immune system.

Astragalus: Increases metabolism, improves immune system, fatigue, heart.

Bilberry: Diabetes, eye conditions.

Butcher's Broom: Circulatory system, e.g. varicose veins and hemorrhoids

Cat's Claw: Anti-oxidant, anti-infection, high anti-inflammatory, blood pressure.

Chamomile: Often brewed as a tea, chamomile can help to reduce the cramping symptoms of menstruation, gas, and other digestive upsets.

Dill: Anti-inflammatory.

Echinacea: Anti-viral, anti-fungal, anti-bacterial.

Elderberry: Anti-viral.

Fenugreek: Stabilizes blood sugar, aids digestive tract, reduces cholesterol.

Ginkgo Biloba: Memory, ADD, circulation, depression, blood pressure, impotence, PMS, tinnitus, stroke, eyes, headache, vertigo.

Ginseng: Stress, immunity, fatigue, asthma.

Green Tea: Cancer prevention, cardiovascular system, digestive system, tooth decay, weight loss.

Licorice: Reduces fatigue, immune system, digestive tract, adrenal glands, liver, anti-inflammatory, asthma, reflux, shingles.

Milk Thistle: Detoxifies the liver.

Olive Leaf: Anti-viral.

Saw Palmetto: Baldness, prostate, bladder infection.

St John's Wort: Depression, anxiety, anti-virus, S.A.D., cream for injuries.

Stevia: Natural sweetener.

SUPPLEMENTS

A healthy body given good nutrition does not generally need drugs and, with a few exceptions, does not need supplements. Some people take dozens each day, but they are not a "magic bullet" and you can't expect to keep eating a SAD diet and make up for it with supplements. It is best to rely primarily on plant food for micronutrients, particularly since that is essentially the only source of phytochemicals. But as we get older, the body becomes less able to assimilate nutrients, so supplements may become more necessary. Consider a Multi-vitamin to replace nutrients depleted from the soil, DHEA and CoQ10 as you age, Fish oil for the brain and general health, and Vitamin-D3 unless you get a lot of sun. For inflammation—an issue for most people—add Astaxanthin. Total: About 50 cents a day.

Science believed for a long time that DHEA, produced by the adrenal glands, is simply a useless hormone, as the appendix is a useless organ. They couldn't find a purpose for either. Studies showed that DHEA is always high in youth and, beginning about age thirty, goes down as we weaken with age, until it is near zero at death, but pharmaceutical science insisted that was just a coincidence. No link could be proven, and drugs were marketed to treat all the symptoms associated with aging. Stephen Cherniske and others demonstrated, however, that the body synthesizes other hormones from DHEA, including testosterone and estrogen. It also influences more than 150 metabolic functions and has substantial effects on many characteristics associated with youth. It is a "trigger" that signals the body to maintain itself at certain levels of strength, energy, and vitality. Muscle mass, bone density, weight control, inflammation, immunity, Alzheimer's, Parkinson's, energy, mood, memory, decision-making, sleep, and energy are all related to DHEA levels. When older people exercise with little improvement and continual injury, it is due primarily to low DHEA. DHEA is also important to brain function, and it has been found that the brain manufactures its own. After Cherniske published *DHEA Breakthrough*, the drug industry tried four times, unsuccessfully, to push a Bill through Congress banning DHEA. Their motive? As with many things, follow the money trail.

Coenzyme Q10 (CoQ10) is produced by the body and found in every cell. It begins to diminish after about age 20 and is low in people on prescription drugs or with chronic diseases, including heart disease, Parkinson's, cancer, diabetes, and HIV. It is oil soluble and is said to be "vitamin-like" because the FDA decided all vitamins had been identified before this one was discovered. It is an antioxident and is important to cell growth and maintenance but, most importantly, it is involved in 95% of energy production. It is highest in organs using a lot of energy, such as the heart.

Supplements are a $25 billion industry in America and many are worthless and even dangerous, particularly some of the over-hyped "patent medicine", weight loss, and energy products. Even good supplements may react adversely with pharmaceutical drugs. Consumer Reports specifically found the following available supplements to be dangerous (To make it more difficult to avoid them, they are marketed under many names): Aconite, bitter orange, chaparral, colloidal silver, coltsfoot, comfrey, country mallow, germanium, greater celandine, kava, lobelia, and yohimbe. There are many other toxic supplements, as well as toxic versions of good supplements. The Chinese have proven time and again that they have no interest in quality and will sell anything Americans can be induced to buy. Avoiding their products, however, is no guarantee, as they provide many of the raw materials used by domestic supplement manufacturers. As an example, fish oil in capsules may contain toxins and is frequently rancid. (Poke a hole in a capsule and smell it.)

Do not take any supplement unless you understand exactly what you expect it to do, are certain what is in it, have thoroughly researched each of the ingredients, know the source is reliable, and have ascertained the supplement is in a form usable by the body. Multi-vitamins should be whole-food based and chelated minerals are often more absorbable. ("Chelation" combines the mineral with an organic molecule, such as a protein, that substantially increases absorption.)

With books and the internet, it is relatively easy to determine what is available, compare prices, and find reports, both for and against, for careful evaluation. If there are no reports, or reports only from the manufacturer, avoid the product. Closely observe any apparent effects of any supplement used. Just because a particular supplement does not seem to work, however, does not necessarily mean your body doesn't need it. You may have obtained an ineffectual brand or are using a supplement that is best used in a combination, which your research should disclose.

The following is a list, in alphabetical order, of some good basic supplements. Most herbs can also be obtained as supplements.

AAKG: A compound of the amino acids L-arginine and alpha-ketoglutarate that promotes circulation and vasodilation. It increases oxygen supply and nutrient delivery to muscles. It stimulates production of human growth hormone (HGH).

Acetyl-L-Carnitine: An amino acid that assists with a host of conditions, including cardiovascular, energy production, diabetes, etc., etc. It assists in carrying fats thru cell membranes for energy.

Adrenal Extract: Supports the adrenal glands. Combats allergies, arthritis, autoimmune disease, lower back pain, and fatigue.

Aloe Vera: Internal (with aloin removed) or topical for wounds, burns, sunburn, and GI tract.

Apple Cider Vinegar [Use with canola oil and spices in salad dressing]: Blood pressure, obesity, arthritis, osteoporosis, leg cramps, diabetes, fungal infections.

Astaxanthin: A derivative of algae, it is among the most powerful combinations of anti-oxidant and anti-inflammatory.

Brewer's Yeast: Assists in diabetes, fatigue, and cholesterol. High selenium.

Colloidal Silver: Potent anti-bacterial in cream or tincture.

Cordyceps: Antioxident, builds the immune system.

CoQ10: Antioxident, energy, cardiovascular health.

Curcumin (in Turmeric): Found in curry. Powerful anti-oxidant, anti-inflammatory, and anti-infection. Similar effects to astaxanthin.

DHEA: Everyone should consider taking this hormone as they become older. A derivative, **7-KETO**, shares many benefits and is not subject to overdose, so it is advantageous to take, along with moderate amounts of DHEA.

Enzymes [Many]: Catalysts in metabolism that affect all cell functions and are critical to immunity. Many supplements are compounds of several.

Fish Oil: Richest source of omega-3 fatty acids DHA and EPA. Strengthens the immune system and vascular system, fights inflammation and many diseases, including cancer, cardiovascular disease, diabetes, high blood pressure, etc., etc. It is important to brain health.

Flaxseed Oil: Similar to fish oil, except it lacks DHA, which is most important.

5-HTP: Synthesizes seratonin, a mood enhancer. For anxiety, depression, food cravings and weight loss, insomnia, headache, S.A.D.

Glucosamine+chondroitin: Arthritis, sprains.

Glutathione: The antioxident in all cells, it is synthesized by the body from anti-oxidant foods. Health can be gauged by the percentage that is reduced (opposite of oxidized), with an ideal ratio of 90%. It fights many diseases, including aging, cancer, Parkinson's, AIDS, and fatigue. It is not well absorbed as a supplement, so it is best to eat many fruits and vegetables to obtain it. Asparagus is highest. SAMe, melatonin, whey protein, and alpha-lipoic acid are its precursors and V-D3 increases brain levels.

Grapeseed Extract: An antioxident. For microcirculation, skin, joints, ligaments, tendons, blood vessels.

Grapefruit Extract: Anti-fungal, anti-bacterial. For sinusitis, IBS.

Kelp: Rich in iron and minerals. For anemia and hypothyroid.

L-Arginine. An amino acid. A strong vasal dilator and important to immunity and healing. Lowers blood pressure. Best taken with L-citrulline.

Lycopene: A carotenoid from cooked tomatoes and other sources. For atherosclerosis, cancer, immunity, macular degeneration, prostate.

Lysine: An amino acid the body does not synthesize. Found in legumes, grains, and meat. Aids cold sores, osteoporosis, and shingles.

MCT: (Medium-chain triglycerides, 9 fatty acids). Energy, athletic training, diabetes, hypothyroid.

MSM: Allergies, arthritis, asthma, inflammation, hair and nails, headaches.

Pectin: Diabetes, cholesterol. Provides fiber.

Perilla Oil: High in alpha linolenic acid. Cardiovascular, inflammation, brain function, allergies, arthritis, memory, nerves.

Phenylalinine: An amino acid. Depression, lower backpain, arthritis, Parkinson's, pain.

Potassium: Blood pressure, heart.

Probiotics: Good bacteria for the gastro-intestinal tract, with a substantial boost to the immune system. Combat cancer, IBS, allergies, etc. A good probiotic will have bifidobacterium, lactobacillus, and other forms of beneficial bacteria.

Progesterone: Menstrual cycle and other female issues, PMS, osteoporosis, autoimmune diseases.

Psyllium: Soluble fiber. Constipation, diarrhea, IBS, diabetes, diverticulitis. Including fiber from food, the body should have 25 grams daily.

Rhodiola Rosea: Mental clarity, stress, energy, immunity, skin condition, depression (increases seratonin and dopamine).

Royal Jelly: Fatigue, cholesterol, stress.

SAMe: Arthritis, depression, fibromyalgia, detoxification.

Selenium: cataracts, depression, cancer, heart, hypothyroid.

Shark Cartilage: Inflammation, arthritis, cancer.

Vitamin B Complex: Metabolism, skin, muscles, immunity, and cell growth. Deters pancreatic cancer if ingested as food.

Vitamin C: Immunity, healing, muscles, and joints.

Vitamin D: Immunity, osteoporosis, cancer, cardio-vascular disease. Almost everyone in America is deficient. Take D3

Hormones are not nutrients from food but are chemicals produced by cells that affect other cells. In effect, they act as chemical messengers.

Hormones have long been used as medicines. A blood, urine, or saliva test may be used, if indicated, to determine if they are within proper range. A "natural" hormone is identical to that produced by the body; a "synthetic" hormone may be produced in nature but is not completely identical. Most are available only by prescription, including insulin, thyroid, estrogen, testosterone, and growth hormone. The following are available as supplements over-the-counter.

Hormone	Typical Dose	Function	Natural Source	Toxic if O.D?
DHEA	10-25 mg	Aging, Inflammation, immunity, libido, healing, metabolism, cognition, mood, muscles, weight, etc.	Adrenal glands, brain	Minor
Melatonin	.5 mg	Aging, jet lag, insomnia, cancer	Pineal gland	Y?
Pregnenolone	10-50 mg	Arthritis, depression, memory, psoriasis	Adrenal gland	N?
Progesterone	Varies	Female issues, osteoporosis	Adrenal, ovaries, brain	N

Enzymes are protein-based substances synthesized in or by the body that act as catalysts in metabolism. There are many of them and they fight infection, inflammation, and diseases such as cancer and autoimmune diseases. They are critically important to digestion, nutrient absorption, vision, hearing, smelling, breathing, organ function, and removal of toxins. They are best obtained from a healthy digestive system and from fresh fruits and vegetables, raw, as cooking destroys them. There are no enzymes in refined or processed foods and freezing reduces them. Supplements are available, if indicated, and it is best to choose one with a broad range of enzymes in an enteric-coated tablet, to avoid destruction by stomach acid. Common enzymes include the following:

Enzyme	Function	Natural Source
Ptyalin	Starch into sugar	Salivary glands
Amylase	Starch into sugar	Pancreas
Pepsin	Breaks down proteins	Stomach
Protease	Break down proteins	Gut bacteria
Lipase	Breaks down fats	Pancreas
Trypsin	Peptides into amino acids	Pancreas
Sucrase	Breaks down sucrose	Small intestine

| Lactase | Breaks down lactose | Small intestine |
| Maltase | Breaks down maltose | Small intestine |

A PLAN FOR GOOD HEALTH

Good health begins with good nutrition, but changing a lifetime of poor diet habits is made even more difficult by a society that will do everything it can to thwart you. Advertising, government recommendations and requirements, food in grocery stores, restaurant menus, and even friends will try to encourage and coerce you into maintaining a SAD diet of excess meat, sugar, refined grains, processed foods, and toxins. For good health, youthfulness, energy, and longevity, consider developing and practicing the following Six-step Program. It will inhibit disease and can often reverse it. Working together with family and friends, for mutual support and information exchange, can be very helpful. Perfection is not required, but as you work at it and feel better you will be encouraged to push farther toward good health habits:

One: Journal. Depending on issues and goals, it may be helpful to keep a journal of your health or weight-loss program in a small notebook. The following sections could be included:

Goal: Dr Amen suggests starting with a *detailed* description of your goal, your motivation, what you expect success to do for you, and your plan to reach the goal. It is a contract with yourself. Note beginning weight and, if weight loss is in the program, your target weight, including milestone goals. Read the goal section every morning, if helpful to maintain focus on your plan for the day. People often sacrifice long-term goals to an immediate urge, and a daily reminder helps keep you centered.

Issues: List any particular health issues you want to address and what you hope to achieve for each.

Good Foods: List the foods and types of foods that fit your health or weight-loss program and the amount of water you will drink.

Bad foods: List the foods and toxins you specifically need to avoid.

Supplements: After careful research and consideration, list supplements you will take, how much, and the purpose for each. Leave space for modifications as your program progresses.

Log: Each day, to the extent you think is helpful, list the foods eaten for breakfast, lunch, dinner, and snacks and a check to show physical exercise, brain exercise, enough water, and supplements. If your program includes weight loss, calorie counting is not important—the real issue is what you eat, not how much. Make weekly notes of progress in weight loss (if applicable), issues, and anything else relevant.

LOG

(Date)	B'fast		Lunch	
	Dinner		Snacks	
	Supplements?	Exercise?	Brain Exercise?	Water?
	B'fast		Lunch	
	Dinner		Snacks	
	Supplements?	Exercise?	Brain Exercise?	Water?
	B'fast		Lunch	
	Dinner		Snacks	
	Supplements?	Exercise?	Brain Exercise?	Water?
	B'fast		Lunch	
	Dinner		Snacks	
	Supplements?	Exercise?	Brain Exercise?	Water?
	B'fast		Lunch	
	Dinner		Snacks	
	Supplements?	Exercise?	Brain Exercise?	Water?
	B'fast		Lunch	
	Dinner		Snacks	
	Supplements?	Exercise?	Brain Exercise?	Water?
	B'fast		Lunch	
	Dinner		Snacks	
	Supplements?	Exercise?	Brain Exercise?	Water?
Weekly Progress:				

Two: Toxins. Begin your health program with a good cleanout and stop ingesting poisons! Are these things worth destroying your health? This includes caffeine, "energy" drinks, alcohol, tobacco, chlorinated water, avoidable food additives, diet soda, and any over-the-counter or prescription drugs you can do without as your health improves and your immune system becomes stronger. These toxins are highly oxidative and inflammatory and they lower DHEA levels. Read labels; it will surprise you what has been hidden in so-called "health foods". The average life expectancy for men in Utah, even though only half are Mormon and not all of them follow the health law, is a full ten years longer than the rest of America. Toxins damage your liver, which has to filter them, your GI tract, which provides 80% of your immune system, your brain, and all other organs and systems. *The Detox Strategy*, by Brenda Watson, provides several stages of detoxification, from a simple system to use periodically to a complex system that really gets your body cleaned out, including heavy metals such as dental mercury.

Three: Nutrition. Stop eating a SAD diet. Excess meat, refined grains, refined sugar (of which the average American eats nearly one hundred-fifty pounds per year!), fast food, processed food, overcooked food, saturated fat, and soda destroy your body and pack on weight. They are not only low in nutrition, they are high in calories, oxidants, and inflammatories. To ensure a balanced diet of macronutrients, enough fiber, and enough micronutrients, eat primarily natural, healthful foods. Include *real* whole grains, (which are high in protein and micronutrients), including 100% whole wheat bread and pasta and brown rice, and enjoy lots of fruits, vegetables, herbs, and spices, which are virtually the only source of phytochemicals. Drink at least eight glasses of water each day. Unsugared lemon water is a good choice. The Bible tells of the capture of Israel about 600 B.C. by Nebuchadnezzar. Daniel and three others were taken captive to the King's court to be trained, and were offered a rich diet, which was thought to be the most healthful—probably similar to an American diet, high in meat and refined foods. They declined. After only a month of the self-discipline of simple food, they were healthier and their skin and hair were noticeably better than those who ate the King's fare.

Four: Supplements. Supplements should be used judiciously. Though many look for an easy way out, they are not a substitute for a nutrient-rich diet and they provide only a few phytochemicals. It is not good to glut on a cocktail of likely-looking products, but carefully consider what you may need and do further research in books and online to make well-reasoned personal decisions. Supplements are natural products but can have profound effects on the body. If used improperly or in improper combinations with pharmaceuticals, they can be injurious. It is also easy to get started and go way overboard, so keep it simple and if something isn't working stop using it.

Basic supplements are important, however, to replace nutrients that are generally lacking, needed as we age, or indicated for individual issues, such as genetic concerns or temporary conditions. Consider especially the four areas of oxidation, inflammation, infection, and stress and determine any that need particular attention. Consider the following possibilities for a basic program:

Multivitamin. This is intended to provide basic nutrients, including those that have been depleted from the soil. Look for primarily V-B1, B2, B6, B9, V-C, V-E, zinc, copper, magnesium, manganese, selenium, and chromium.
DHEA. This hormone is more and more important after about age 30, as the adrenal glands slow down. Overdose causes acne on men and facial hair on women. A blood test can show actual level.
CoQ10. It is responsible for 95% of energy, as well as many other functions, but starts to decrease after age 20.
Fish Oil. Best source of Omega 3. It is anti-inflammatory and contains many micronutrients. Not only good for the body, it is good for the brain, and can help counteract many of the issues and diseases of aging.
Vitamin D3. Most Americans are deficient. It is important to immunity, absorption of calcium, prostate health, and other issues. Recent studies have shown that cancer increases with distance from the equator, and Vitamin D

not only reduces the chance of cancer, it can arrest it. (Multi-vitamins don't typically have enough. Overdose can cause kidney damage and several lesser problems, but it takes a *lot*.)

Astaxanthin or **Curcumin**. These are probably the most effective natural combination anti-oxidant and anti-inflammatories. Dr Oz recommended astaxanthin as the #1 supplement.

Calcium+Magnesium+Zinc. Particularly, though not only, for older women.

Glucosamine+chondroiten. If you have joint problems. An anti-inflammatory is needed to allow it to reach injured cells.

Herbs and Spices. For micronutrients, use lots. For example, **Turmeric**, the principle ingredient in curry, is a super antioxident, anti-inflammatory, and immunity builder. **Garlic** is good for the cardiovascular system. You don't have to actually eat the nasty stuff, it comes in "odor-free" pills. **Onion**, unfortunately, has essentially the same benefits—and disgusting characteristics—as garlic, but also can be taken as a pill. **Cinnamon and Honey** (unpasteurized) are particularly good in combination and defend against infection, cardiovascular disease, cholesterol, arthritis, colds, flu, upset stomach, hearing loss. They help youthfulness, the immune system, and weight loss. Honey does not cause blood sugar spikes.

Probiotics. For GI health, these should be taken periodically.

Five: Exercise. Bodies are efficient and will only develop the capacity demanded of them—use it or lose it. With DHEA, CoQ10, proper diet, and moderate exercise, muscles will be developed and used, resulting in calorie burn and the message to the body to build itself and to turn from storing energy to using it. Energy level will increase dramatically and living will become much more pleasurable. Studies show that even the brain grows as a result. Lack of exercise reverses this process quickly.

Most of us know we don't exercise enough. But exercise takes so much time and is totally boring! Not with *The Exercise Advantage* (Section 2). It takes minimum time and is effective and comfortably progressive, even for those who have not exercised in many years. A Norwegian study showed that women who exercise are 62% less likely to develop cancer.

The Exercise Advantage was inspired by the old 11-minute Canadian Air Force 5BX exercises, but three newer exercises, suggested by a professional trainer, are safer. An additional four minutes of recommended stretches are advisable, particularly as muscles shrink and stiffen with age. The program is adapted for men (including older boys), women, and elementary-age children. It will take a month or so for inactive people to become re-accustomed to exercise, and in a month the exercise habit will be established. Your body will begin to feel better, you will have more energy, and substantial progress will provide motivation to continue.

Six: Sleep. Almost half of Americans do not get proper sleep, six-to-eight hours, and chronic sleep loss is a major factor in stress. It suppresses the immune system and the libido and can lead to many illnesses, including hypertension and heart disease. Insomnia has many causes, including lack of certain substances, such as melatonin, DHEA, and V-B12, use of stimulants, eating at bed time, breathing problems, and interruption of circadian rhythms by failure to develop habitual sleep patterns. Individual circumstances should be analyzed and addressed, and supplements are available to assist with natural sleep. Pharmaceuticals are not recommended.

DIGESTIVE HEALTH

Toxins play a far more destructive role in health than most people realize. Beginning in the womb, our bodies carry varying amounts of 700 toxins. They are created through the normal processes of metabolism, they are a major component of a SAD diet, they are in air, water, plastics, cosmetics, clothing, buildings—the list is nearly infinite—and many people are voluntarily addicted to substances containing them. Some morbid person did a study that showed our bodies, after death, decompose more slowly than in the past, as a result of the preservative nature of all these chemicals.

The World Health Organization claims that 85 of 102 major diseases, covering the alphabet from allergies to stroke, are caused or exacerbated by toxins. To reduce exposure to toxins, it is important to breathe clean air, drink filtered water, avoid chemicals, including common ones like cosmetics, pharmaceuticals, and household products, avoid mold, and avoid caffeine, alcohol, tobacco, and artificial sweeteners (agave, stevia, and honey are best).

Chemicals in plastics, such as BPA (bisphenol A), dioxins, and pthalates, are carcinogens and can enter food when microwaved or wrapped in plastic. A Harvard study found 69% more BPA in urine of adults who drank from BPA-based plastic bottles. An American Medical Association study linked high levels of BPA with heart disease and diabetes. BPA also acts like estrogen and has been linked to hormonal irregularities, premature menopause, and possible infertility. The numbers 2, 4, or 5 in the triangle on the bottom of a container mean no BPA.

Our bodies have seven systems for elimination of toxins and waste products, including blood, lymph, kidneys, lungs, skin, liver, and colon. There are 100 trillion bacteria in the GI system (as compared with 10 trillion cells that compose the human body). Some are pathogenic, some neutral, and some beneficial. For good health and a strong immune system, it is necessary to maintain a proper ratio, about 4–1, between good and bad bacteria, as they have several functions, including aiding digestion, maintaining a healthy intestinal lining, and strengthening immunity. They provide 80% of the body's immune system. On three levels, different strains of friendly bacteria attack toxic microbes, viruses, and other substances: As they pass thru the intestinal tract, as they attempt to penetrate the intestinal lining, and after they have passed through the lining. A cold, for example, is not just the result of exposure, but a breakdown of the bacterial immune system. Many conditions, even very serious ones, that seem entirely unrelated to digestion are, in fact, simply the result of an imbalance or reduction of good bacteria.

Six major enemies attack the friendly bacteria in the digestive system: 1] Antibiotics. They destroy both good and bad bacteria, but the bad bacteria recover more quickly and get out of balance. Even if you don't take antibiotics, they are in all animal products. 2] Pathogenic microbes. Yeast is the most common—there are far worse ones—and they multiply rapidly if good bacteria are reduced. 3] Antacids. Continual use is destructive of bacteria and, ironically, people who take antacids are just as likely to be suffering from inadequate acid, as symptoms are the same. Acid is not only necessary to digestion, it is the first line of defense against biological toxins. 4] Undigested food. Reduced acid contributes to this, as does inadequate chewing and insufficient levels of digestive bacteria. Bad bacteria thrive on fermenting food, especially meat, and inflammation of the GI tract follows. 5] Toxins. This includes all those we are exposed to in modern life and the ones people voluntarily ingest, such as drugs and coffee. Sugar kills good bacteria and feeds bad bacteria. 6] Aging. Bifida bacteria are particularly reduced as people age. It is important to supplement these, as they are particularly important to digestion and immunity. Unprocessed fermented foods, including sauerkraut and yogurt, are often high in probiotic bacteria, though many commercially-available yogurts are high in sugar and low in probiotics.

For good GI health, it is important to minimize toxins and, particularly as we age, to take probiotic bacterial supplements to maintain the ratio. The two most prevalent good bacteria are Lactobaccillus, in the small intestine, and Bifidobacterium, in the large intestine. These bacteria thrive on fiber, which is one reason it is so important. When selecting a probiotic supplement, it should have five strains of each bacteria, have a bacteria count of 15 billion per serving by the expiration date, and be delay-release, such as an enteric-coated or bio-tract tablet, so it will not dissolve in the stomach where acid will kill the bacteria.

Along with immunity, aging, and appearance, the digestive system also directly affects weight loss. Poor elimination causes water and fat retention, interferes with metabolic and elimination processes, and inhibits glucose from getting into cells, resulting in reduced energy, increased fat storage, and inflammation. All cells of the body can store toxins, but fat cells are the primary location, which sets up a vicious cycle of increasing toxins and increasing fat.

In addition to taking probiotics, regular cleanout of the digestive system helps keep it healthy. Intestines can store some awfully rude stuff, causing partial blockage, inflammation, and other issues, and they need to be flushed out. Otherwise, IBS, acid reflux, diverticulitis, and other conditions, including cancer, can develop. Fasting regularly, e.g. monthly for 24 hours, is helpful as it rests the digestive system and helps it purge itself. Once a year, for up to 3 days, take only soluble and insoluble fiber, Aloe-vera, watermelon, prune juice and other juices, lots of water, and heavy doses of V-C. On completion, take probiotics to replace good bacteria.

The Detox Strategy, by Brenda Watson, recommends maintaining a healthy GI system by taking plenty of water and fiber, basic supplements, periodic use of probiotics, and four levels of cleanout to neutralize toxins and develop a healthy digestive system. Level 1 is a 2-week basic cleanout, involving soluble and insoluble fiber, nutrition and supplements, that should be done up to twice a year. Level 2 is an advanced cleanout that can be done less frequently, as needed. Level 3 is specifically for the liver, and is a one-time, or at least infrequent, cleanout for those who have particular liver issues, including people who intentionally ingest toxins, such as alcohol or caffeine. Level 4 is specifically for removing heavy metals, such as mercury from dental fillings. A long list of herbs is provided for each cleanout, with a suggestion that supplements be found with as many of them as possible. You can check supplement sources for ingredients of their detox kits or go on Brenda's website.

BRAIN HEALTH

The human brain is the most complex thing in the universe, and has more synapses (connections) than there are stars! Brain health is complex, but it is as critical to aging as is the health of the rest of the body. Dr Daniel Amen, MD, PhD, a psychiatrist and researcher who specializes in physical and mental diseases of the brain, has done SPECT brain scans of 60.000 healthy and unhealthy brains. Unhealthy brains look like Swiss cheese—black holes for all the dead sections of the brain where blood no longer flows. Genetics and aging are factors, but the worst damage is from alcohol, caffeine, smoking, illegal drugs, and toxic fumes. Fortunately, however, scans show that brain cells can be partially regenerated with proper treatment. Long believed impossible, the brain can grow new cells, as well as adapt for dead ones by growing new synapses among existing cells.

After years of research and practice, Dr Amen has learned that many psychological and physical illnesses are often best treated with nutrition rather than drugs, though diagnosis and medication by a doctor who specializes in nutrition may be needed. These include ADD, OCD, sociopathy, depression, bipolar disorder, panic attacks, anger, aggression, Parkinson's, suicide, and Alzheimer's, which can be at least delayed, if caught early. A program to protect and repair the brain includes:

- Protect it physically. It is the consistency of jello, and easily damaged.

- Quit poisoning it with toxins and drugs. Smoking and more than 2 glasses of wine per week or 1 cup of coffee per day damage the brain. Is brain damage worth the antioxidant properties of wine? There are better ones.
- Get proper diet. Include 1] plant proteins, 2] complex carbs, such as blueberries, broccoli, decaf green tea, oatmeal, oranges, spinach, and nuts; 3] good fats, particularly fish oil; 4] take supplements, including vitamins, antioxidants, anti-inflammatories, and iron, if anemic.
- Drink lots of water; at least two quarts a day.
- Get proper sleep.
- Exercise your brain: Learn something *new* every day—work it *hard* for 15 minutes.
- Exercise your body: Aerobic workout that requires coordination and sweating is particularly good for the brain, e.g. table tennis.
- Avoid ANTS (automatic negative thoughts). These actually have a physiological effect on the brain that is cumulative. Each day, write down five things you're thankful for.
- Have sex three times a week (if appropriate). In addition to brain health, it also reduces chances of heart attack by 50%.

WEIGHT CONTROL

Diets don't work. Despite the irony of $40 billion spent annually on dieting by desperate Americans, two-thirds remain overweight and half of those are obese. Studies show diets have a 95% failure rate, as weight loss is almost inevitably followed by weight gain—and the gain often exceeds the loss. It has a terrible effect on self esteem as well as health, as it builds up more internal fat. Paradoxically, weight control is primarily *not* a matter of counting calories or a question of self-discipline—fighting to stay on a diet—it is an issue of metabolism, and it gets worse with age. Eat less, exercise more *does not work*, it just creates muscular fat people. As with poor health, weight problems are exacerbated by—more accurately, caused by—the SAD American diet. So forget the scales and counting calories and focus instead on eating healthful, nutrition-rich food instead of unhealthful, calorie-rich food. If you live a healthy lifestyle, weight loss will follow automatically, together with better health, more energy, and increased resistance to disease. A SAD diet encourages acidity, so start by maintaining a proper alkaline state that reduces the body's need to grow fat cells. For example, drink lots of lemon water which, paradoxically, helps contribute to a state of alkalinity.

Most popular diets fall into one of four classes: Low protein/high complex carb, low carb/high protein, low fat, and low calorie. A study showed that each worked equally well for weight loss—in the short term—but none worked for most people in the long term. They can also have serious adverse consequences for health. Diets are catabolic, nutrient-poor, and sacrifice long-term health to short-term weight loss. As nutrients and energy are reduced, total metabolism is reduced by as much as 30%. The body goes into survival mode, living off muscle tissue and actually increasing fat-storing enzymes. This even continues for up to six months after the diet is discontinued, which explains subsequent weight gain. Muscle reduction results in even lower requirements for energy, so even more food is stored as fat. The immune system is also damaged by lack of nutrition and the aging process is accelerated, as the body does not receive the raw materials necessary to reproduce healthy cells.

A new Harvard study (based on twenty years of data involving nearly half a million people) showed they gained an average of 18 pounds over the period and that weight gain is determined more by quality than quantity of food eaten. The worst foods are potatoes (probably because they tend to be eaten in large amounts), particularly chips and french fries, soda (which also destroys calcium), red meat, and processed meat. Also high on the list are refined grains, sugary foods, and alcohol. The best foods for minimal weight gain are yogurt, vegetables, fruit, nuts, and whole grains. Paradoxically, the more people eat of these foods, the less weight they gain. Lifestyle is also important. Those who exercise—surprise!—gain less weight. Those who sleep less than six or more than eight hours or who watch a lot of TV also gain more weight.

Insulin levels are key to both weight control and health, and refined sugar and grains need to be shunned like the plague. A blood sugar spike, from eating sugar or refined foods, causes insulin to be produced, insulin causes cells to store calories (as fat), blood sugar plummets, hypoglycemia and fatigue kick in, setting off hunger signals, and you start looking for another sugar hit. Periods of high insulin levels reduce DHEA and white blood cells and encourage hypertension, heart disease, and diabetes. Toxins like caffeine, alcohol, tobacco, and legal and illegal drugs also need to be avoided.

Recent studies have examined two types of muscles: "fast twitch" and "slow twitch". Fast twitch muscles, for strenuous exercise, use sugar (glucose) for fuel; slow twitch muscles, for endurance, use fat. It was observed that exercises that strengthen slow twitch muscles develop many and larger mitochondria in cells, which enhance fat burning. They looked for a drug that could increase the production of mitochondria without exercise, by tricking the body into thinking it was low on fat fuel so it would develop mitochondria. They developed "Aicar". Ten days of inactivity results in muscle atrophy equal to 15 years aging! (a compelling reason to exercise regularly), but Aicar allowed couch potato mice to run 44% farther with no exercise. They also lost weight. No tests have yet been performed on humans. (Probably no difficulty finding volunteers!) In the meantime, endurance-building exercise is vital to burning fat.

The China Study Plan for weight loss is based on research for *The China*

Study, which demonstrated that, in addition to its major health effects, a primarily plant-based diet is most effective for weight control, both immediate and permanent. To lose weight, eat all you want of whole, *unrefined* plant foods (precluding white flour, sugar, white rice, refined pasta, etc) and substantially reduce animal products. For good health, avoid toxins like caffeine, tobacco, and alcohol and eat a minimum of animal products, though there is no need to obsess about strict compliance. If this plan is followed temporarily, as a weight-loss diet, it will work temporarily; it needs to be adopted as a permanent change in lifestyle. It will be initially difficult, not just because of changes in habits but also because we are actually addicted to unhealthful foods. It will take a real commitment of several weeks to overcome the addiction as well as develop new habits. You will probably feel sick and rundown for an initial period and want to quit and go back to the old habits. But there is a healthy reason for feeling ill: it is called withdrawal. You will soon feel so much better.

A plant-based diet encourages anabolic metabolism, healthy cell reproduction, and good health, emphasizing proper and sufficient nutrition at the cellular level. Reduction in body fat is merely a healthy side effect, as calories are converted into energy used in the anabolic process. This is no quick fix: it took a long time to put it on, and will take a while to get it permanently off. Although people frequently lose up to 10-17 pounds the first month, a continuing weight loss of about one pound per week can typically be expected. It will also stay off, as the body becomes more and more healthy, thermogenic (heat-producing), and *younger*. Weight will stabilize as ideal weight is achieved. You will never have to count calories again.

Dr Amen's Plan is based on his studies of brain health and his findings that nutrition and supplements are generally more effective than medication for treating both physical and psychological brain conditions. They also do not have bad side effects. Fortuitously, as his patients followed his recommendations for a healthy brain, he discovered they also developed a healthy body—and lost substantial weight! He now advises patients to eat whole grains and a large variety of fruits and vegetables, while avoiding tobacco, caffeine, alcohol, drugs, sugar, refined grains, and processed foods. He discovered that obesity actually shrinks the brain and advises patients not to be a dinosaur: large body, small brain, and early extinction! Supplements he recommends specifically for losing weight include fish oil, V-D, Chromium, alpha-lipoic acid, and, depending on body type, SAMe, 5-HTP, St John's wort, or green tea; one of which should help reduce food cravings.

Dr Fuhrman's Plan is based on his career as a medical doctor working in the wellness field, helping patients overcome disease through nutrition. His book *Eat to Live* proves the success of his program and details his research, case studies, a plan for a healthy lifestyle, and a collection of nutritional, palatable recipes. The program includes a 6-week introduction followed by a lifetime plan, based on a food pyramid he developed. Unlike the now-discredited food pyramid pandered through the U.S. Government by the meat and dairy industry, which suggested up to 35% animal protein, Fuhrman's pyramid provides, from the base upward:

1] 30-60% vegetables, half of them raw and half of them cooked. They can be eaten in unlimited quantities and you will still lose weight if starchy vegetables are limited. The main meal each day should be a large salad with many different vegetables.

2] 10-40% beans, legumes, and at least four fruits each day.

3] 10-40% seeds, nuts, avocadoes, whole grains, and potatoes (with grains and potatoes in the minority).

4] Less than 10% poultry, oil, eggs, fish, and fat-free dairy.

5] Beef, cheese, sweets, and processed foods eaten rarely.

The book provides dozens of case histories of the success of the program, both for reversal of serious diseases and invariable weight loss. One-pound-per-day weight loss can be expected for two weeks, followed by slower, but consistent, loss until ideal weight is stabilized. One hundred pounds or more in a year is frequently accomplished. Fuhrman recognizes that perfection is essentially unobtainable, but the greater the compliance, the better the effects. Obviously, compliance to any reasonable degree is better than a SAD diet.

Dr Fuhrman's six-week plan overcomes food addictions, initiates detoxification, and builds momentum for weight loss. It provides for eating three meals a day, all you want but no snacks, of: 1] Raw vegetables (at least 1 pound) and cooked nutrient-rich vegetables, such as mushrooms, peppers, eggplant, onions, tomatoes, carrots, broccoli, cauliflower; 2] Legumes, including beans, bean sprouts, and tofu; 3] At least 4 fruits daily; 4] A maximum of 1 cup per day of the following: Cooked starchy vegetables, whole grains, squash, corn, white potatoes, sweet potatoes, brown rice, or whole grain bread or cereal; 5] A handful of raw nuts and seeds, particularly including flaxseed. Off limits are: Animal products, including dairy, sugar, processed foods, fruit juice, snacks, and oils. Fuhrman provides two weeks of recipes that support this plan. Salad is the main dish, with Fuhrman's own high-nutrient, low-calorie dressing.

Fuhrman's permanent plan provides for an all-you-can-eat diet of 90% plant-based foods, allowing for 10% processed and animal-based foods, up to 2 servings daily, and an occasional "falling off the wagon". By comparison, the SAD diet is composed of 62% processed foods and 26% animal products.

Cherniske's Plan is an alternative, if you still insist on going on a "real" diet. The following healthful weight-loss plan is a synopsis from *The DHEA Breakthrough*:

- Gradually reduce calories, to avoid initiating starvation mode. Never eat fewer than 1200 calories per day, with supplements to ensure adequate nutrition.
- Eat more frequent, smaller meals. This does not mean graze all day long! Never go for an extended period without a meal. Skipping breakfast, particularly, puts the body in starvation mode, slowing down metabolism and increasing fat storage. Sumo wrestlers use this technique to put on massive amounts of weight! They fast, then gorge and take a nap. Sound familiar? Americans also eat far less healthful food than Sumo wrestlers.
- Eat plant protein and *complex* carbohydrates. Limit fats, as they can easily be converted directly into body fat, rather than going through an energy-burning process to be converted. Unsaturated fats, in moderation, are healthful—fish oil, olive oil, canola oil, safflower oil, nuts.
- Eat many different kinds of fruits and vegetables. They all have different nutrient combinations.
- Avoid diet products, including diet calcium-destroying soda. They have few calories, but are loaded with toxins.
- Engage in strength-training exercise a few times each week and get at least moderate cardio-vascular exercise each day, e.g. walking. It signals the body that it needs to turn food into energy, not fat, as well as building muscles that use calories. The only way to get rid of fat is for the body to burn it, which requires an efficient oxygen system..
- Do not use food as a substitute or crutch when angry, alone, or bored.
- Have healthful alternatives available for snacks, such as carrots, celery, or fruit.

Some supplements suppress appetite; perhaps as the body gets nutrients it needs, it stops sending extraneous hunger messages. Eat your main meal at breakfast, for energy through the day, and a light meal at dinner, as sleep is disturbed while digesting, and sleep is critical. The following supplements may be particularly helpful to weight control:

Bioenergetics. CoQ10, chromium, and alphaketogluteric acid improve energy and insulin metabolism.
Cactus. Prickly Pear cactus has traditionally been used in Mexico and South America to treat diabetes. It modifies blood sugar levels and sends glucose to the brain without triggering an insulin reaction. It helps maintain a positive mood and a clear head, even on reduced calories.
Fiber. A teaspoon of fiber with a glass of water before each meal maintains a feeling of fullness. It is also healthful.
5-HTP. Reduces cravings for sweets and improves mood by increasing seratonin.

Garcinia Cambogia. Helps control appetite and decreases conversion of calories to fat. Be sure it contains 50% HCA, to be effective. It is best taken between meals, 2 or 3 times a day.

L-glutamine. Reduces appetite.

MCT Oil. Medium chain triglycerides are fats that go directly into the bloodstream and, even in small amounts, provide energy and inhibit fat storage by the body.

Probiotics. A healthy GI tract is necessary for efficiency of all metabolic functions.

Protein. To control appetite, take a small amount of a simple protein supplement, e.g. peptide, with a glass of water 20 minutes before main meals. It stimulates CCK hormone in the small intestine, decreasing appetite.

Astaxanthin. In a study, 12-18 mg per day for 12 weeks lowered belly fat.

All these programs share a common theme: By eating a primarily plant-based diet, restricting animal protein, weight loss is unavoidable—with side effects of increased energy and good health. By sticking with it, you overcome addiction to a SAD diet and begin to enjoy foods that are actually healthful. Self discipline is always a problem. Keep only healthful foods around the house—so you have no choice! Though calorie counting is not the key to weight loss, comparing different foods should provide motivation to get healthy nutrition. For example, lettuce has 7 grams of fiber, 0 fat, and 65 calories per pound. Sirloin steak has 0 fiber, 11 grams of saturated fat, and 850 calories per pound. A little scary.

Whatever plan you choose to follow, it is important to identify healthful, primarily plant-based, foods that you really like. Eating unsatisfying foods can be counterproductive to weight control, as more is eaten in a vain attempt to be satisfied and the plan is finally discarded. Mouths are not garbage disposals—so slow down and enjoy it! Studies show that inadequately chewed food, particularly meat, ferments in the gut, causing toxins and disease. Time spent eating affects level of satisfaction, sense of fullness, and amount eaten. For complete nutrition, take the basic supplements listed in "A Plan for Good Health".

NATURAL REMEDIES

Healthful nutrition and basic supplements will take care of most symptoms by creating a healthy body. This is a condensed list of specific supplements for common ailments, developed by many societies over, sometimes, thousands of years. It is a place to start your personal research. Review specific issues and check other resources, such as books or online, for full information.

Acid Reflux

Licorice, aloe vera, nux vomica, slippery elm, probiotics.

Allergies
V-C, stinging nettle, MSM, quercitin, fish oil, flaxseed oil, thymus, probiotics, protease enzyme. For itching, take as hot a shower as possible to neutralize hystamines.

Alzheimer's / Dementia / Memory Loss
DHEA, huperzine, rhodiola, niacinamide, astaxanthin, fish oil, acetyl-L-carnatine, DHA, vegetable oils, sage, ginkgo biloba, club moss, phospatidylserine, V-B12 [for myelin], V-E, bacopa, choline, folic acid, V-C, lecithin. Early signs of Alzheimer's include difficulty smelling strawberries, pineapple, lemons, and natural gas. Obesity, smoking, inactivity, depression, and high blood pressure greatly increase the risk.

Anti-oxidants
Astaxanthin, spices such as cloves and turmeric, nuts, fruits, vegetables, beans, and berries such as cranberries and blueberries. Unsweetened chocolate scores high.

Anti-inflammatories
Astaxanthin, aspirin, ibuprofen, V-A, V-C, V-E, fish oil, olive oil, peanut oil, canola oil, cat's claw, proteolytic enzyme, and selenium. Fruits, nuts, and vegetables are often anti-inflammatory. A Mediterranean diet is highly anti-inflammatory. Although natural fish is anti-inflammatory, farm-raised fish is inflammatory. Sugar, caffeine, and other toxins are highly inflammatory.

Anti-infection
Good nutrition and reducing oxidation and inflammation are the first line of defense. Good oral hygiene is extremely important. Turmeric, olive leaf, cranberry juice, and oregano fight infection.

Anti-stress
Ginseng, St John's wort, L-tyrosine, eleuthero root, lemon balm. Exercise, deep breathing, meditation, self-discipline, better sleep, and laughter.

Anxiety and Panic Attacks
Often as simple as dehydration, so drink water. Avoid acidic foods: Meat, sugar, refined foods, nots, and grains. Eat alkaline foods: Vegetables and fruits, including citrus (paradoxically, it is alkaline in the body). Take flaxseed oil, V-B complex, adrenal concentrate, colloidal minerals, potassium, and gatorade.

Arthritis
Glucosamine-chondroiten, astaxanthin, niacinamide, pregnenolone, MSM, fish oil, protease enzyme, cayenne, cayenne cream, V-C, V-D, SAMe, melatonin, 5-HTP, selenium.

Back Pain
MSM, calcium/magnesium, astaxanthin, protease enzyme, glucosamine, cayenne cream, V-C, V-D, V-B complex. Avoid inflammatory food: sugar, refined grain, caffeine, etc. Exercise.

Bladder Control
Pumpkin seed, ginseng, valerian root, cornsilk, magnesium. Kegel exercise any time you're sitting, and hold it longer. Bladder capacity can't be increased, but strengthening the muscles helps.

"Body Blues"
A condition, particularly in women, of chronic irritability, fatigue, overeating and insomnia. Each day, get as much light as possible, 20 minutes outdoor exercise, and a multivitamin with B-1,2,6,9 V-D, and selenium. Improvement after 2 months.

Burns, including sunburn
Aloe vera cream, ice or ice water, coat with flour, cantharis, L-glutamine, zinc, bioflavonoids, fish oil, V-C, calendula, carotenoids, antioxidents. Avoid sugar.

Cancer
V-C/D/E, astaxanthin, betacarotene, selenium, coriolus versicolor, maitake, proteus enzymes, astragalus, turmeric, curcumin, essiac, fish oil, calcium, carotene, garlic, cranberries, rosemary, folic acid. Avoid animal products. Saturated fats increase risk and accelerate cancer growth, as do infection, acidity, and inflammation. Dairy products increase mucus, which cancer feeds on. There are claims that asparagus can arrest cancer, as well as kidney stones and other diseases. It has been found to be high in several potent anti-cancer micronutrients and is the highest in glutathione. Four tablespoons twice daily of a puree of cooked asparagus is recommended.

Cardiovascular Disease
DHEA, Garlic, CoQ10, fish oil, hawthorn, magnesium, ginkgo biloba, L-carnitine, V-E, V-C, cayenne. Avoid animal protein.

Carpal Tunnel
V-B6, bromelein, glucosamine, boswellia, calcium+magnesium, ginkgo biloba.

Cholesterol
Take garlic, fish oil, antioxidants, guggul, V-C, V-B-complex, V-E, soluble fiber with lots of water, beta-carotene. Exercise. Eat fruits, vegetables, oatmeal (not instant), olive oil, canola oil, spices, red grapefruit, pecans, almonds. Avoid meat, trans fats, and saturated fats, e.g. butter.

Cold Sore
Most important: maintain a strong immune system. Take L-lysine, zinc, V-B complex, and C. Eat broccoli and cabbage. Avoid L-arginine and foods rich in it, such as meat and dairy products.

Common Cold
V-C, hot peppers, zinc, ginger, astragalus, oregano, garlic, thymus.

Cough
Buckwheat honey.

Depression

DHEA, rhodiola, pregnenolone, V-D, SAMe, 5-HTP, St John's wort, ashwaganda, V-B complex (esp. niacinamide), fish oil, ginkgo biloba, L-tyrosine, L-tryptophan, SAMe, 5-HTP, St John's wort, B-complex, potassium, calcium/magnesium, zinc, phosphorus. Avoid caffeine, sugar, salt.

Diabetes

Fiber, fish oil, V-B complex, V-C, V-E, pancreus extract, magnesium, chromium, copper, CoQ10, brewer's yeast, soy, garlic, bilberry, gymnema sylvestra, alpha lipoic acid, vanadyl sulphate, cinnamon, evening primrose oil, prickly pear. Avoid caffeine, alcohol, saturated fat, sugar, refined foods, milk.

Digestive Disorders and IBS

Fiber, aloe vera, probiotics, ginger root, peppermint oil, raisins. Juice-fast regularly. Avoid caffeine, alcohol, refined sugar and retined grain. May be caused by a wheat allergy. Corn syrup for constipation.

Ear Infection

V-C, V-A, fish oil. Dissolve a garlic pill or St John's wort in warm water or oil and irrigate ear canal.

Energy builders

CoQ10, whole grains, DHEA, V-B complex, MCT oil, acetyl-L-carnitine, alphalipoic acid, alphaketogluteric acid, Astragalus, Ashwaganda, folic acid, chromium, phosphorus, manganese, Alpha lipoic acid, potassium, and magnesium aspartate. Exercise.

Fatigue

DHEA, CoQ10, kelp, fish oil, V-B complex, V-C, magnesium, cordyceps, NADH, L-carnatine, ginseng, malic acid, licorice, peppermint, move around.

Gout

Half-pound cherries and 1 quart cherry juice, fish oil, flaxseed oil, chlorella, bromelain, folic acid, with capsicum cream applied topically. Check pH level for acidity. Eat berries, nuts, seeds, soy, and soluble and insoluble fiber, to eliminate acidity and uric acid. Drink lots of water. Use only mono- or poly-unsaturated fats and avoid sugar and refined grains. Do a thorough GI tract detox with a 3-day juice fast and cleanout, with a supplement "kit", followed by several days of probiotics and eating lots of raw fruits and vegetables.

Hair Loss

(May be caused by pharmaceutical drugs) Saw palmetto, fish oil, biotin, MSM, silica, molasses, V-B complex V-C, V-E, zinc, rosemary oil shampoo. Avoid refined hydrogenated oil, sugar, and grains.

Headache

Magnesium, V-B2, V-B6, 5-HTP, parthenolides, fish oil, melatonin, flaxseed, calcium+magnesium, lots of water. Eat onions, brussel sprouts, garlic, and broccoli. Avoid sugar, coffee, alcohol, refined grains, dairy products, and very cold drinks.

Hearing Loss

Ginkgo biloba, V-B complex, esp.12, V-E, cayenne, garlic, bromelein.

Heart Disease
Mayo Clinic: Exercise; avoid tobacco, alcohol, meat, and dairy products; take fish oil; eat whole grains, fruits, and vegetables; lose weight; keep cholesterol and blood pressure down. For heart attack: put 2 aspirin under the tongue and do not lie down. Symptoms include: Severe pain in chest, left arm, or chin. Women are often different: Extreme fatigue, weakness, dizziness, cold sweat, shortness of breath, anxiety.

Hemorrhoids
Fiber with lots of water, berries, flax oil, bilberry, butcher's broom, horse chestnut, collinsonia, grapeseed extract, aloe vera juice, V-C, probiotics.

Hypertension
Potassium, calcium+magnesium, CoQ10, garlic, fish oil, hawthorne, V-C, argine, pomegranate, rosemary, hawthorne. Reduce sodium.

Hypoglycemia
A diet of whole foods, avoiding refined grains, processed foods, and sugar. Multi-vitamin, including V-B complex.

Hypothyroid
Iodine, V-E, taurine, forskolin, ATP. Avoid sugar, soy, and stress.

IBS
Fiber (not wheat bran) with lots of water, probiotics, aloe-vera, peppermint. Avoid sugar, coffee. Complete a cleanout. IBS may be caused by parasites or liver disease.

Impotence
DHEA, L-arginine, cordyceps, ginseng, ginkgo biloba, ptency wood, puncture vine, niacin, zinc. Avoid caffeine and alcohol.

Insomnia
Calcium+magnesium+zinc, V-B complex, magnesium, exercise. Before bed: melatonin, 5-HTP, chamomile tea, peppermint, nutmeg, passionflower, valerian, hops, corydalis. A shower at bedtime is relaxing and clears sinuses.

Kidney Stones
Cranberries, aloe vera, pumpkin seeds, juniper berry tea, magnesium, V-A, V-B6, V-C, V-E, IP-6, boron.

Leg Spasms
CoQ10, V-D, V-E, lots of water.

Macular Degeneration.
Astaxanthin, lutein, zeazanthin, betaine hydrochloride, zinc, ginkgo biloba, bilberry, flavanoids, fish oil, V-E, carotenoids, selenium, grapeseed extract.

Menopause
DHEA, V-E, calcium/magnesium, valerian tea, black cohosh, progesterone cream, vitex, ginseng, hops, rehmenia, soy protein.

Motion Sickness
Ginkgo biloba, V-B complex, magnesium, cocculus. Before the event, try:

Ginger, peppermint, cinnamon, black horehound, tabacum.
MS
DHEA, fish oil, V-B12, V-E complex, plant sterols and sterolins, probiotics, GLA, (numerous others for specific symptoms).
Muscle Aches
Calcium/magnesium, potassium, homeopathic magnesia phosphorica, MSM, V-B complex, protease enzymes. Quinine water for leg cramps.
Osteoporosis
DHEA, gelatin, calcium+magnesium, boron, V-B complex/C/D/K, zinc, manganese, ipriflavone, fish oil, soy protein. Test for acidity and eat an alkaline diet. Avoid soda.
Pain relief
White willow bark, MSM, SAMe, fish oil, V-B complex, V-D. turmeric, proteolytic enzymes, bananas [including skin lining], avoid sugar, refined grain, caffeine, saturated fats, and other inflammatories.
Parkinson's
DHEA, CoQ10, V-C, V-B complex, fish oil, calcium/magnesium, NADH, NAC, dopamine agonist, menocycline, creatine. Eat protein later in the day.
pH Balance
Eat fruits and vegetables, reduce sugar, meat, and dairy. Paradoxically, drink lemon or lime water. Take calcium+magnesium but *do not* take antacids!
Prostate
Tomatoes, fish oil, V-D, pygeum, zinc, garlic, onions/chives, citrus, saw palmetto, pygeum africanum, glutamic acid, rye pollen, nettle, beta-sitosterol, amino acids. soy, pumpkin seeds, exercise.
Seasonal Affective Disorder
St John's wort, melatonin, SAMe, 5-HTP, V-B complex, folic acid, selenium, fish oil, ginkgo biloba, amino acids, V-D, light therapy, exercise.
Shingles
Homeopathic rhus toxicodendron, V-A, V-B12, V-C, V-E, Capsaicin cream [or eat lots of hot sauce], licorice, lysine, olive leaf extract, echinacea, zinc.
Sinusitus
N-acetylcysteine, bromelain, grapefruit seed extract, colloidal silver, V-C, grape seed extract, garlic, turmeric, echinacea, oregano, elderflower tea, anti-fungal: flaxseed, quercitin, pro-biotics, N-acetylcysteine, saline rinse, horseradish.
Skin
Fish oil, flaxseed oil, rosemary, rhodiola, V-B comples, probiotics, silicon, alfalfa, grapeseed. Avoid sugar and toxins like caffeine and nicotine.
Sprains
Bromelain, glucosamine, MSM, V-C, boswellia, arnica, fish oil, aspirin or ibuprofen, silica.
Stroke Prevention and Recovery

According to the Mayo clinic, stroke prevention is the same as heart disease prevention: Garlic, fish oil, canola oil, policosanol, V-C, V-E, ginkgo biloba, calcium, green tea, cayenne, cinnamon, ginger. Avoid meat and dairy. To diagnose stroke: Can speak O.K., lift both arms above head, smile evenly on both sides? Stroke Risk (3 checks): Blood pressure over 140/90; Cholesterol LDL over 100, HDL under 50; Diabetes or blood sugar over 100; Smoke; No regular exercise; Family history of stroke.

Tinnitus
Astaxanthin, magnesium, zinc, choline, V-B12. May be a symptom of hypertension.

Thyroid
DHEA, bladderwrack, chromium, thyroid glandular, pituitary glandular, L-tyrosine, progesterone, gugul, thyroidinium, fish oil.

Vision
Fish/flaxseed oil, astaxanthin, carotenoids, lutein, zeazanthin, betaine hydrochloride, zinc, ginkgo biloba, bilberry, flavanoids, V-E, selenium, grapeseed extract, V-A [night vision]. Work through the attached eye chart a few times a day.

PAIN RELIEF
The problem of pain is illustrated by the fact that Americans spend $6 billion per year for relief. Serious pain is of two kinds, acute (severe) and chronic (long-term). Although, it is often possible just to "buck up" temporarily for acute pain, chronic, relentless pain can be devastating and needs serious treatment. Natural remedies to reduce pain and promote healing, including supplements, are often at least as effective as pharmaceuticals, have fewer side effects, are not addictive, and do not cause stomach problems or cardiovascular risk. V-D deficiency, a condition with most Americans, has been associated with chronic pain, requiring a double dosage of painkillers. Relaxation therapy, music, and exercise can be helpful. Conversely, lack of activity, such as long periods sitting at a desk, increase pain. A daily 30-minute walk is often a good pain reducer.

For both immediate and long-term relief, it is important to reduce inflammation. It exacerbates pain and inhibits proper nutrients from getting into the cells, preventing the body from repairing itself. Inflammation is a body defense to injury or disease and should end when the condition is healed. It may continue, however, and specific remedies may be necessary to get rid of it. Anti-inflammatory supplements are available, but equally important is a non-inflammatory diet, high in micronutrients and low in animal products, fats, sugar, caffeine, tobacco, and alcohol. All these increase inflammation and pain.

There are many remedies for pain and here are some that have been found effective:

Acetyl-L-carnitene+alpha-lipoic acid can ease nerve pain and regenerate damaged nerves over time.

Arnica, from a European flower, is available as an ointment for topical use or as a pill to hold under the tongue, up to six times daily. It has been found helpful in reducing the pain associated with joints and muscles.

Aspirin, Acetaminophen, and **Ibuprofen** can be helpful for pain and inflammation if not overused. Overuse can cause serious and sometimes irreversible disease, including diabetes and liver damage.

Astaxanthin, from algae, is a powerful anti-inflammatory and anti-oxidant.

Calcium+magnesium+zinc supplements have been found effective in reducing the pain and stiffness of arthritis. Up to 2400 mg a day of a supplement such as Aquamin is recommended.

Capsaicin, the "active ingredient" in hot peppers, can be eaten or applied as a cream one to four times daily. Like an anesthetic, it acts by deadening pain receptors. One study showed arthritis users reduced pain by half with topical application for a month and neuropathy patients achieved the same result after two months use. Migraines were substantially reduced by application inside the nostrils.

Curcumin, a powerful anti-inflammatory, is found in **turmeric**, the main ingredient in curry. It is available as a supplement and studies have found it helpful for arthritis and psoriasis. It can be taken four times daily, along with taking fish oil and avoiding animal fats.

Fish oil, high in Omega-3, in doses of 1000–4000 mg per day can be somewhat effective in reducing pain. It is more effective with 1000 units of **V-D** and 2-4 g of **DHA+EPA**, especially for arthritis and autoimmune diseases. Fatty foods and Omega-6 should be avoided.

Heat and **Ice** are often effective pain relievers. Topical application of ice within 48 hours of injury is recommended, followed by heat in the morning, such as a hot soak, and ice in the evening. **Massage** can also be helpful.

MSM has been shown to reduce arthritis pain and increase physical function after three months, particularly if used with glucosamine. Start with 1.5–3 g daily and increase to 3 g twice daily if pain persists.

REM sleep reduces pain and increases healing, as well as relieving depression. If pain is severe, sleep may be difficult, but every effort needs to be made to get 6-8 hours sleep each night. Narcotic painkillers prevent REM sleep, setting up a vicious cycle of pain, requiring more and more painkiller and leading to addiction.

SAMe is made in the body from an amino acid and is available as a supplement. It is a strong anti-inflammatory and increases seratonin and dopamine levels. In one study, it reduced arthritis pain by 50 percent after two months and had no side effects of conventional medications. 400–1600 mg daily is recommended, together with **turmeric** and **fish oil**. It can interact negatively with pharmaceuticals, particularly antidepressants, and is not for people with bipolar disorder. It is expensive and degrades if exposed to light.

VISION

How's your vision? Is it getting worse with age? Are you squinting as you try to focus?

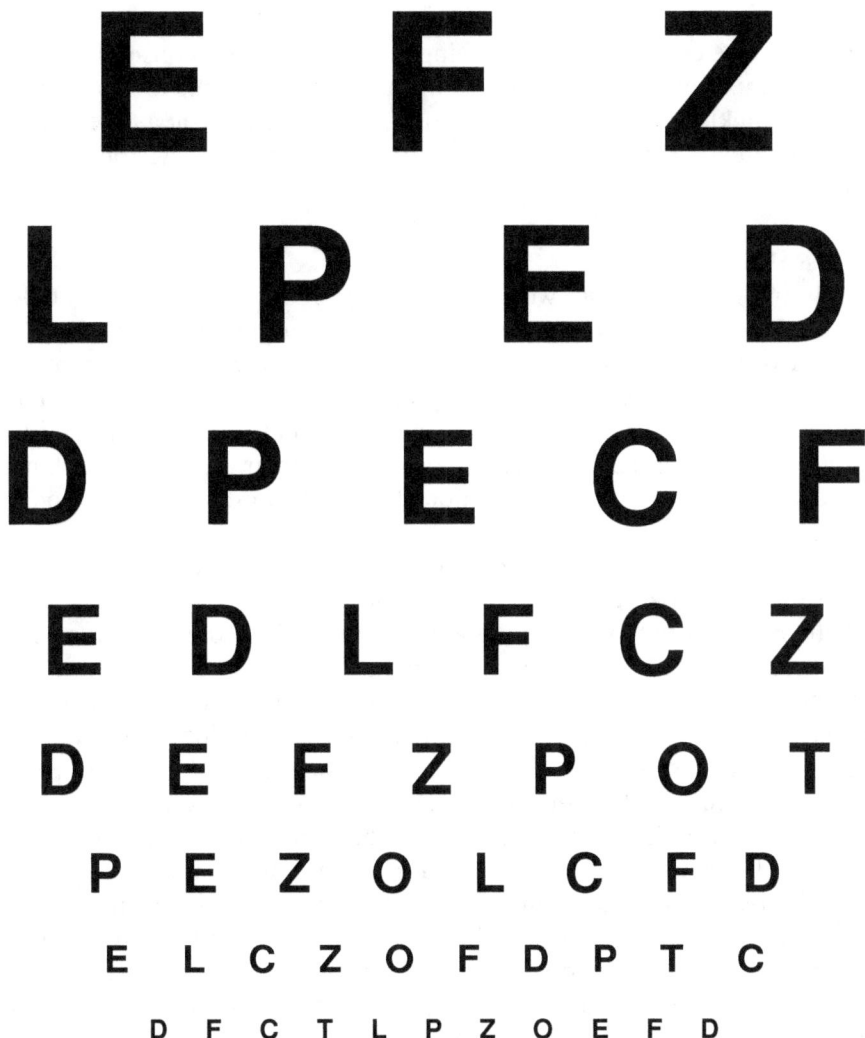

Focusing becomes more difficult with age, as the cornea becomes less flexible. Nutrition, particularly carotenoids, and supplements may help, with V-A for night vision. It has been proven in studies that using glasses causes the eyes to gradually worsen, requiring ever-stronger lenses. Wear magnifiers for several minutes, then take them off and see what has happened to your vision. On the other hand, personal experience has shown that vision can often be improved by exercise that forces the cornea to change focus, such as working with an eye chart a couple times each day. The medical profession has recently begun using temporary eye patches to help the other eye improve.

To use an eye chart, set the page as far away as you can read line three easily. Begin at the top, focusing on each feature of each letter and slowly tracing the outline with your eyes as you work your way down the page, one eye at a time.

Another eye exercise, used by racing drivers, is to focus on something very close, within several inches, and then instantly change focus to something at a distance, quickly switching back and forth. Again, one eye at a time. Do each of these exercises a couple times a day for a week and see if vision does not improve.

RECIPE IDEAS

Food is important and, as well as providing good nourishment, should be enjoyed. Many view eating a plant-based diet as a great sacrifice, but that is not necessarily so. In a carnivorous society, few have explored the possibilities of flavorful and satisfying plant-based recipes. A creative vegetarian cookbook is a good start—and be grateful you don't need to go entirely to that extreme! Be careful, though. With their fixation against animal products, vegetarians seem much more lenient toward processed foods and refined grains, such as bagels, one of the most oxidative foods there is. Dr la Puma's *Book of Culinary Medicine* is a great resource for foods and good recipes that target particular health conditions.

Withdrawal symptoms from the addiction to a SAD diet can be overcome by several weeks of maintaining a primarily plant-based diet and avoiding junk food. You will then feel better and look better, and the new diet will become comfortable and satisfying. Since good health does not require total abstention, an occasional steak, for example, is entirely appropriate. Because it is not frequent, it will be enjoyed even more. The same is true of *occasional* desserts loaded with sugar and calories. They will, however, probably taste too rich and sweet and more moderate desserts will be desired.

Food is expensive and getting more so. Spices, for example, are prohibitive at grocery stores if, as recommended, many are used. Bulk food stores are a much better alternative, particularly if larger amounts of foods are purchased. Online can be a good source. For example, 50# of TVP (textured vegetable protein, from soy) was bought for $60, including shipping. It is reconstituted 3-1 with water or bouillon. It is high in protein and in many recipes is interchangeable with ground beef. It can also be given various meat flavors.

From simple fare to gourmet creations, choices are up to your taste, creative ability, and willingness to put out the effort. Just remember to cut way back on animal products, saturated fat, refined grains, processed foods, and sugar. Add as many spices and herbs as possible, for flavor and micronutrients. Eighty percent of taste is smell, so emphasize it for satisfying meals. Here are a few suggestions, just to get started.

Breakfast

Eat protein, preferably from plants, such as legumes, soy, or whole wheat, for a long-term energy source.

Hot cereal of oatmeal, cracked wheat, or brown rice. Preferably no milk, except soy or almond milk. Add fruit, such as raisins or dates, vanilla, ground cinnamon or cloves, and a little sea salt. Sweeten with honey and cinnamon or stevia.

Fruit and nuts.

Pancakes, waffles, or crepes of whole-wheat flour. Mix in mashed banana, berries, chopped nuts, or shredded coconut. For topping, have honey, fruit run in the blender, or a pate' of a fruit such as apples, pears, or peaches with dates, nuts, cinnamon, and a pinch of ginger, run in the blender.

Lunch

A large green salad, with a variety of vegetables, is an obvious choice. Don't put 400 calories of fatty dressing on a 60 calorie salad. A dressing of apple cider or balsamic vinegar with olive or canola oil and lots of herbs and spices is good.

Fruit salad made from a variety of available fruits. Add some vanilla and cinnamon for enhanced flavor.

Vegetable-based soup with whole-grain bread.

Dinner

There are any number of recipes made without meat, refined grains, or processed foods. Most recipes that can be made with ground beef can use TVP. Possible dishes include stew, soups, chili, brown rice pilaf, spanish rice, whole-grain pasta with marinara sauce, nachos, and tacos.

Sausage is made with some or all the following spices, which can be combined and kept to mix with water to reconstitute TVP, e.g. for sausage gravy: 1 1/2 tsp salt, 1 tbs fresh black pepper, 1/2 tsp cloves, 1 tbs sage, 1/4 tsp cayenne pepper, 1 tbs garlic salt, 2 tbs chopped rosemary, 3 tbs chopped marjoram, 1 tbs red pepper flakes, 2 tbs fresh coriander seed, 6 tbs honey, 2 tbs celery salt, 2 large ground bay leaves, 1 tsp thyme, 1 tbs oregano, 2 tbs parsley, 1/2 tsp allspice, 2 tbs crushed fennel seed, 1 tsp paprika.

Desserts

The important thing is to cut way back on sugar, refined grains, and unhealthy or excess oils and fats. The English say that Americans stop at the candy store, buy one pound of candy to take home—and eat the whole thing. Anything worth doing is worth doing to excess, right! The English, on the other hand, carefully select *one* confection to take home and leisurely enjoy. Some dessert possibilities include:

Stewed Fruit, with sliced apples, pears, or peaches, chopped dates, 2 tbs honey, 1 tbs ground ginger, ½ tsp cardamom, 1 tsp cinnamon, and 2 cups water. Blend about 1/3 of the mixture, stir it back in, and cook in a saucepan. To bake as a crisp, use whole wheat flour.

Tapioca Pudding, with coconut milk and stevia or honey.

Coconut Balls, with 2 cups shredded coconut, 4 ripe mashed bananas, ¼ cup cocoa powder, and 1 cup chopped nuts (optional). Blend ingredients, form into small balls, and bake at 350 for 20 minutes.

Rice Pudding, with pre-cooked brown rice, mashed ripe banana, 1 tsp cinnamon, ¼ tsp nutmeg, stirred together with a little water and baked at 350 for 20 minutes.

Fruit Kabobs, with cut-up fruit marinated in apple juice with cinnamon, nutmeg, or other spices, skewered, and baked or broiled on a pan coated with non-stick spray.

Smoothie, with 1 scoop pre-sweetened (with stevia) vanilla whey protein powder, ½ cup water, ½ cup ice, run in the blender with blueberries, banana, or other fruit. Or use chocolate powder with peanut butter or mint.

REFERENCE SOURCES

Information in this Section is based substantially on review and synopsis of many books and other sources. The following are particularly recommended. Information in this book has not been evaluated by the Food and Drug Administration and is not intended as medical advice or to diagnose, treat, cure, or prevent any disease. Consult with your own health care practitioner for individual medical recommendations. The information concerns dietary supplements, over-the-counter products that are not drugs.

THE CHINA STUDY, by T. Colin Campbell, PhD.
EAT TO LIVE, by Joel Fuhrman, M.D. [Everyone should read this.]
CHANGE YOUR BRAIN, CHANGE YOUR LIFE, by Daniel Amen, M.D.
THE DETOX STRATEGY, by Brenda Watson, N.D., C.N.C
STOP PAIN, by Vijay Vad, M.D.
NATURAL CURES, by James Balch, M.D. and Mark Stengler, N.D.
THE DHEA BREAKTHROUGH, by Stephen Cherniske. M.S.
THE METABOLIC PLAN, by Stephen Cherniske. M.S.
ChefMD BOOK OF CULINARY MEDICINE, by John la Puma, M.D.
DEARPHARMACIST.com, by Suzie Cohen. Many excellent health articles.
Wikipedia. Lots of information on most every subject.
Online supplement sources, with information: puritan.com, vitacost.com, renewlife.com, purecaps.com, sourcenaturals.com

THE BOTTOM LINE

Good nutrition is key if you want the best chance of looking and feeling younger, of having more energy and brain capacity, of living free of disease, and of avoiding doctors and drugs. The goal is not perfection but, to cut to the chase in a complex subject, keep these simple principles in mind:

- *Carbs*: Eat *real* whole grains and many varieties of vegetables and fruits. Drastically reduce sugar, refined grains, and processed foods.
- *Proteins*: Maximize proteins from plants, including legumes, whole grains, and brown rice. Substantially reduce meat and dairy.
- *Fats*: Eat small amounts of olive oil, safflower oil, canola oil, and a handful of nuts daily.
- *Water*: Drink at least 8 glasses—2 quarts—of filtered lemon water a day, for hydration, to flush toxins, and to help maintain an alkaline pH balance.
- *Supplements*: Regularly take Multi-vitamins, DHEA, CoQ10, Fish or flaxseed oil, V-D3, Astaxanthin. Add any that address specific issues.
- *Spices*: For micronutrients, use lots of different herbs and spices, especially turmeric, ginger, oregano, and cinnamon with honey.
- *Toxins*: Shun coffee, tea, alcohol, tobacco, unfiltered water, diet products, food with additives, and other toxins of modern society.
- *Dieting*: If weight is a problem, choose one of the plant-based diet programs that is also good for health and permanent weight loss.
- *Snacks*: Have healthful alternatives, such as fruits, carrots, and celery.
- *Cleanout*: Take a thorough cleanout to start, fast monthly for 24 hours, and take a cleanout annually. Follow each with probiotics.
- *Hygiene*: Wash hands often and brush teeth (and tongue) and floss.
- *Activity*: Engage daily in both physical and mental activities you enjoy, preferably with others who will increase the pleasure and motivation. As a minimum, walking every day is critical.
- *Rest*: Get six to eight hours sleep each night and take time for relaxation and recreation, particularly including socializing.
- *Review*: Keep a simple journal to note progress: How do you feel, what do you weigh? Can you do the physical and mental things you want to do? Do you need to modify diet, supplements, exercise, or other activities?

If that's even too much to remember, just keep a few points in mind:

- **Eat lots of different kinds of vegetables and fruits.**
- **Reduce sugar, animal products, and toxins.**
- **Take fish oil.**
- **Get some exercise.**

After a month or two of trying these four things, you will feel better and may be motivated to review this book, learn more, and push farther.

THE FINAL WORD: THE WORD OF WISDOM

[Italics added] -D&C 89 [1833]

In consequence of evils and designs which do and will exist in the hearts of conspiring men in the last days, I have warned you and forewarned you by giving unto you this word of wisdom by revelation...*adapted to the capacity of the weak and the weakest* of all saints.

...*Strong drinks [alcohol] are not for the belly*, but for the washing of your bodies. *Tobacco is not for the body*, neither for the belly, and is not good for man, but is an herb for bruises and all sick cattle, to be used with judgment and skill. *Hot drinks [coffee and tea] are not for the body* or belly.

All wholesome herbs God hath ordained for the constitution, nature, and use of man—*Every herb in the season thereof, and every fruit in the season thereof*; all these to be used with prudence and thanksgiving.

Flesh also of beasts and of the fowls of the air, I, the Lord, have ordained for the use of man with thanksgiving; nevertheless they *are to be used sparingly*; And it is pleasing unto me that they should not be used, only in times of winter, or of cold, or famine.

All grain is ordained for the use of man and of beasts, to be the staff of life, not only for man but for the beasts of the field, and the fowls of heaven, and all wild animals that run or creep on the earth; (And these hath God made for the use of man only in times of famine and excess of hunger.) All grain is good for the food of man; as also *the fruit of the vine; that which yieldeth fruit, whether in the ground or above the ground—Nevertheless, wheat for man*, and corn for the ox, and oats for the horse, and rye for the fowls and for swine, and for all beasts of the field, and barley for all useful animals, and for mild drinks, as also other grain.

And all saints who remember to keep and do these sayings, walking in obedience to the commandments, *shall receive health* in their navel and marrow to their bones; And *shall find wisdom and great treasures of knowledge*, even hidden treasures; And *shall run and not be weary, and shall walk and not faint*. And I, the Lord, give unto them a promise, that *the destroying angel shall pass by them*, as the children of Israel, and not slay them.

So now you know *what* you need to do and *why* you need to do it. Ball's in your court!

Section Two - THE EXERCISE ADVANTAGE

R C and Brett Copeland 3/08

Many of us feel guilty, and know our bodies suffer, as we don't exercise enough. But exercise takes so much time, requires special equipment, is uncomfortable, and—worst of all—is totally boring! Right? Not any more! Not with *The Exercise Advantage*.

The Exercise Advantage takes minimum time out of a busy day, under twenty minutes, plus any additional walking or jogging you choose to do, requires no equipment, and is effective and comfortably progressive, even for those who have not exercised in many years. Exercises are simple, can be done almost anywhere, and progress is automatically measured. Maybe the best thing is you don't need a gym, and you won't get bored to death! You are finished almost before you realize it. When you reach your target you can do 1-3 [with stretches] one day and 4-6 on alternate days.

Groups, including families, can do the exercises together, even at entirely different levels, since exercises are similar in execution and time. Everyone can simultaneously work at their own level, six days a week, and take a break on Sunday. It will take a month or so for inactive people to become re-accustomed to exercise, and within a month the exercise habit will be established. Your body will begin to feel good, you will have more energy, and substantial progress will provide motivation to continue.

Exercises progress upward on three Charts, with six exercises and ten Levels for each. As you progress, difficulty increases and reps increase, but time remains the same: under 15 minutes a day, even if you include 4 minutes of optional, but recommended, stretches. *Exercise Advantage* was inspired by the old Canadian Air Force 5BX program, but three newer exercises, suggested by a professional trainer, should be safer, and the program should work for men [including older boys], women, and elementary-age children.

The program adapts to individual physical condition by the Level of exercise initially chosen, the rate of progress, and the final holding point. This is your program, so do it the best, most effective way, for you. Do not rest between each exercise, and if an exercise is too difficult to do all the reps correctly, move back one or more Levels. For Exercise 6, running in place, you may substitute walking, a treadmill, exercise bike, jogging, or swimming. To keep track of running paces [each left foot down], set up a row of pennies, and move one for each 100 paces.

"No pain, no gain" is *not* applicable! If there is any question, a doctor should be consulted for a physical before beginning the program. To avoid the possibility of soreness or injury, the first month should be kept easy, with Chart I, selecting a very comfortable Level to start. Do not force it! Fitness takes time—as Aesop illustrated by his fable, in the long run the tortoise *always* beats the hare. Do not do anything that hurts or may cause injury—the progression will get you there, slow and sure and relatively easy.

Advance at your own comfortable rate, following the "Progress Schedule". For each exercise, add the number indicated by "+" until reaching the total number indicated after "→", then move to the next Chart. After progressing to the point you choose, based on your goals, age, and physical constraints, maintain that Level by exercising three times a week.

The Exercise Advantage is designed to get you reasonably fit and keep you there. If you want to get really serious, there is *The Exercise Advantage - Pro*—with four higher Charts. The only equipment required for them is resistance bands, and exercises alternate between upper-body exercises one day and lower-body exercises the next. If you wish—and can cut it— *The Exercise Advantage - Pro* can take you to a fitness level approaching professional athletes.

So don't let excuses stand in your way to better physical health. With good nutrition and *The Exercise Advantage*, you can do it!

THE EXERCISE ADVANTAGE
- CHART I

Varm-up	**2** **Bii 1 Dog**	**3** **Side 1 ridge**
Walk in place briskly 1 minute. [Recommended: Add 4-minute stretch routine.]	On hands and knees, keep abs *tight* [breathe slowly thru chest]. Extend 1 arm and opposite leg. Stretch and hold 2 breaths. Do 3 reps each side. **[Fig. 1]**	On side, supported by one forearm, keep abs *tight* [breathe thru chest]. Raise hips in line, hold 2 breaths. Do 3 reps each side. [Initially do with knees on floor, if necessary.] **[Fig. 2]**
1 or 5 min.	**3 reps**	**3 reps**
:url-up	**5** **Pu hup**	**6** **Run**
On back, hands under lumbar for support, 1 knee bent, abs *tight* [breathe thru chest]. Raise head and shoulders 1 breath, down I breath. **[Fig. 3]**	On stomach. Push-ups on knees, hands just outside shoulders. Women/Kids: Butt over feet, or hands on a chair. **[Fig. 4]**	Run in place 6 minutes [count each left foot down], doing 5 calf extensions [stretch up on toes] each 50 paces. Alt: Walk ½ mile briskly.
6+1→15	**1+1→10**	**100+25→325**

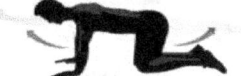 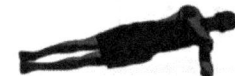

Fig. 1: Bird Dog   Fig. 2: Side Bridge

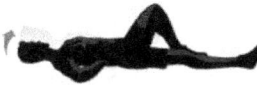

Fig. 3: Curl-up

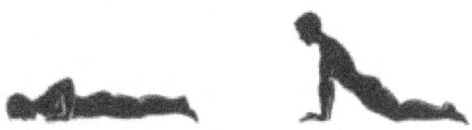

Fig.4: Knee Pushups [For women and kids, raise butt]

PROGRESS SCHEDULE - Chart I

Date	Weight	Level	1: Warmup	2: Bird Dog #Reps [pair]
		1	1 or 5 min.	3
		2	1 or 5 min.	3
		3	1 or 5 min.	3
		4	1 or 5 min.	3
		5	1 or 5 min.	3
		6	1 or 5 min.	3
		7	1 or 5 min.	3
		8	1 or 5 min.	3
		9	1 or 5 min.	3
		10	1 or 5 min.	3

Level	3: Bridge #Reps [pair]	4: Curl-up #Reps	5: Pushup #Reps	6: Run #Reps
1	3	6	1	100
2	3	7	2	125
3	3	8	3	150
4	3	9	4	175
5	3	10	5	200
6	3	11	6	225
7	3	12	7	250
8	3	13	8	275
9	3	14	9	300
10	3	15	10	325

EXERCISE ADVANTAGE – CHART II

1 **Varm up**	2 **Bir 1 Dog**	3 **Side 1 ridge**
Walk in place briskly 1 minute. Raise feet 6 inches. Elbows at right-angle; swing arms. [Recommended: Add 4-minute stretch routine.]	On hands and knees, keep abs *tight* [breathe slowly thru chest]. Extend 1 arm and opposite leg. Stretch and hold 4 breaths. Do 3 reps each side. **[Fig. 1]**	On side, supported by one forearm, keep abs *tight* [breathe slowly thru chest]. Raise hips in line, hold 4 breaths. Do 3 reps each side, rolling on forearms, with body locked, to other side. **[Fig. 2]**
1 min./5 min.	**3 reps**	**3 reps**
:url-up	5 **Pu hup**	6 **Run**
On back, hands under lumbar for support, 1 knee up, abs *tight* [breathe slowly thru chest]. Raise head and shoulders, hold 2 breaths, down 2 breaths. **[Fig. 3]**	On stomach. Push-ups on knees, hands under shoulders. Women/Kids: Butt over feet. **[Fig. 4]**	Run in place 6 minutes. [count left foot down]. Elbows at right angle; swing arms. 10 jumping jacks each 100 paces. Alt: Walk 1 mile briskly.
11+1→20	**11+1→20**	**260+15→395**

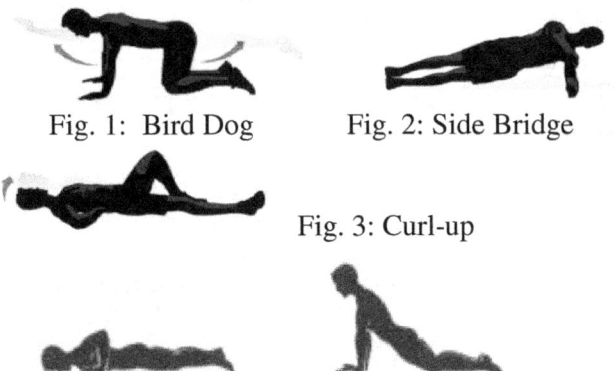

Fig. 1: Bird Dog   Fig. 2: Side Bridge

Fig. 3: Curl-up

Fig.4: Knee Pushups [For women and kids, raise butt]

PROGRESS SCHEDULE - Chart II

Date	Weight	Level	1: Warmup	2: Bird Dog #Reps [pair]
		1	1 or 5 min.	3
		2	1 or 5 min.	3
		3	1 or 5 min.	3
		4	1 or 5 min.	3
		5	1 or 5 min.	3
		6	1 or 5 min.	3
		7	1 or 5 min.	3
		8	1 or 5 min.	3
		9	1 or 5 min.	3
		10	1 or 5 min.	3

Level	3: Bridge #Reps [pair]	4: Curl-up #Reps	5: Pushup #Reps	6: Run #Reps
1	3	11	11	260
2	3	12	12	275
3	3	13	13	290
4	3	14	14	305
5	3	15	15	320
6	3	16	16	335
7	3	17	17	350
8	3	18	18	365
9	3	19	19	380
10	3	20	20	395

EXERCISE ADVANTAGE – CHART III

Warm up	2 Bird Dog	3 Side Bridge
Walk in place briskly 1 minute. Raise knees waist high. Elbows at right-angle; swing arms. [Recommended: Add 4-minute stretch routine.]	On hands and knees, keep abs *tight* [breathe slowly thru chest]. Extend 1 arm and opposite leg. Stretch and hold 6 breaths. Do 3 reps each side. **[Fig 1]**	On side, supported by one forearm, keep abs *tight* [breathe slowly thru chest]. Raise hips in line, hold 6 breaths. Do 3 reps each side, rolling on forearms, with body locked, to other side. **[Fig. 2]**
1 min./5 min.	3 reps	3 reps
Curl-up	5 Pushup	6 Run
On back, hands under lumbar for support, 1 knee up, keep abs *tight* [breathe slowly thru chest]. Raise head, shoulders, and back, hold 3 breaths, down 1 breath. **[Fig.3]**	On stomach, back straight: Men: Push-ups. Women/Kids: Knee pushups,. **[Fig. 4]** Alternate with chair dips	Run in place 6 minutes [count left foot down]. Elbows at right angle; swing arms. 10 "fast feet" [step asap], *and* 10 jumping jacks each 100 paces. Alt: Jog 1 mile.
11+1→20	16+1→25	260+15→395

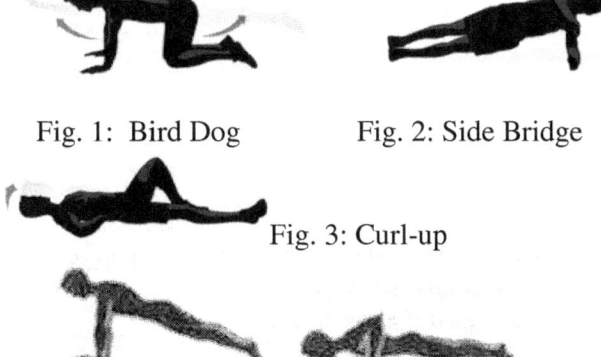

Fig. 1: Bird Dog   Fig. 2: Side Bridge

Fig. 3: Curl-up

Fig. 4: Knee Pushups [Women and Kids]; Pushups [Men]

PROGRESS SCHEDULE – Chart III

Date	Weight	Level	: Warmup	2: Bird Dog #Reps [pair]
		1	1 or 5 min.	3
		2	1 or 5 min.	3
		3	1 or 5 min.	3
		4	1 or 5 min.	3
		5	1 or 5 min.	3
		6	1 or 5 min.	3
		7	1 or 5 min.	3
		8	1 or 5 min.	3
		9	1 or 5 min.	3
		10	1 or 5 min.	3

Level	3: Bridge #Reps [pair]	4: Curl-up #Reps	5: Pushup #Reps	6: Run #Reps
1	3	11	16	260
2	3	12	17	275
3	3	13	18	290
4	3	14	19	305
5	3	15	20	320
6	3	16	21	335
7	3	17	22	350
8	3	18	23	365
9	3	19	24	380
10	3	20	25	395

EXERCISE ADVANTAGE – STRETCHES

Stretches are advised as, along with the running, they develop flexibility and reduce soreness. Do them after Exercise One, Walking in Place. Breathe deeply and slowly while stretching, and count breaths.

1. Stretch side of neck, waist Stretch head and shoulders to one side, as far as possible, turning at waist and neck Hold 3 breaths, then do other side. Repeat two reps	
2. Stretch shoulder and back of upper arm Place right hand over left shoulder Push right elbow across chest above left shoulder Hold 6 breaths. Repeat other side	
3. Stretch triceps, top of shoulders, waist Hold elbow behind head with opposite hand Pull elbow behind head as you slowly lean to side Hold 6 breaths, Repeat other side	
4. Stretch calf Right foot in front, leg bent, left foot behind [or both feet] Move hips forward until you feel stretch in calf of left leg Keep left heel flat and toes pointed straight Hold 6 breaths. Do not bounce! Repeat other side	
5. Stretch front of thigh (quadriceps) Face wall, grasp left foot behind butt with right hand Pull heel toward buttock Hold 6 breaths. Repeat other side	
6. Stretch shoulders, arms, and ankles Lie on floor, arms overhead, legs straight Reach arms and legs in opposite directions Hold 3 breaths, relax. Repeat 2 reps	

7. Stretch side of hips, waist, hamstrings Sit on floor, right leg in front, left foot over right knee Turn head over right shoulder, rotate upper body right Pull left knee toward opposite shoulder Hold 6 breaths. Repeat other side	
8. Stretch back of leg and lower back Bend left leg in at knee Slowly bend forward from hips toward foot of straight leg [Use a towel if you cannot reach your feet] Hold 6 breaths. Repeat other side	

NOTES

Dr Stuart McGill, PhD, has spent 25 years studying and working with professional athletes in all sports. His findings include:

• There are four types of loads on the back: Flexion, shear, compression, and twisting.

• Exercises combining these four loads are particularly deadly and to be avoided.

• The spine is most vulnerable when fully flexed, i.e. bent forward like the letter C.

• Flattening the lumbar curve—the concave segment of the small of the back—is risky.

• Spinal loads of sit-ups, and even crunches, can damage the back.

• The spine is at its strongest in its neutral, S-shaped, position.

• Strength of abs and back is not as important as spinal stability and endurance.

• It is better *not* to have good back flexibility: At the limits of stretch injury can occur.

Dr McGill recommends the Bird Dog, Side Bridge, and Curlup exercises: They build protective strength in the midsection and endurance in the back, while causing minimal stress to the spine. For best effect, brace abdomen for each of these three exercises, as if about to take a punch in the gut.

A short cool-down walk after exercise is also good, as is engaging in various sports and physical activities.

Drink plenty of water.

Acetaminophen [e.g. Tylenol] is reputedly the best pain relief for muscle aches. Recent studies show that taking V-D and avoiding sugar, refined grains, saturated fats, and toxins such as caffeine is effective in pain relief. Astaxanthin is the best natural anti-inflammatory.

THE EXERCISE ADVANTAGE - PRO

For most, *The Exercise Advantage* is more than adequate. For those who have progressed through *The Exercise Advantage* Charts I - III and feel challenged to advance, the following Charts can develop a remarkable level of fitness. Still under 15 minutes a day, four or six days a week, and the only equipment is resistance bands. It will take a few days of practice to get used to these new exercises and get them committed to muscle memory but, with some modifications, they remain the same for all Charts.

EXERCISE ADVANTAGE - PRO – CHART IV

[Exercises are numbered, with their descriptions following the Charts. Stretches are from *The Exercise Advantage*.]

LOWER BODY EXERCISE - Mon., Wed., Fri. [No resistance bands]

1 - Warm up	2 - Hamstring Blasts	3 - Lunges
4 - Calf Extensions	5 - Squats	6 - Run

PROGRESS SCHEDULE– Lower Body Exercises - Chart IV

Date	Weight	Level	1	2	3	4	5	6
		1	3 min.	26	11	16	22	410
		2	3 min.	27	11	17	24	420
		3	3 min.	28	12	18	26	430
		4	3 min.	29	12	19	28	440
		5	3 min.	30	13	20	30	450
		6	3 min.	31	13	21	32	460
		7	3 min.	32	14	22	34	470
		8	3 min.	33	14	23	36	480
		9	3 min.	34	15	24	38	490
		10	3 min.	35	15	25	40	500

UPPER BODY EXERCISES - Tues., Thurs., Sat.
[Use light resistance bands for Exercises 10, 11, 13, 14 15, 16]

1 - Warm up	7 - Bird Dog	8 - Side Bridge		9 - Curl-Up
10 - Tricep Extension	11 - Upright Rowing	12 - Chair Dips	13 - Bicep Curls	14 - Chest Press
15 - Lawn Mower		16 - Forearm Blasts	17 - Pushups	

PROGRESS SCHEDULE – Upper Body Chart IV

	1	7	8	9	10	11	12	13	14	15	16	17
1	3 min.	2	2	11	11	11	11	6	16	11	16	6
2	3 min.	2	2	11	11	12	12	6	17	12	17	6
3	3 min.	2	2	12	12	13	13	7	18	13	18	7
4	3 min.	2	2	12	12	14	14	7	19	14	19	7
5	3 min.	2	2	13	13	15	15	8	20	15	20	8
6	3 min.	2	2	13	13	16	16	8	21	16	21	8
7	3 min.	2	2	14	14	17	17	9	22	17	22	9
8	3 min.	2	2	14	14	18	18	9	23	18	23	9
9	3 min.	2	2	15	15	19	19	10	24	19	24	10
10	3 min.	2	2	15	15	20	20	10	25	20	25	10

EXERCISE ADVANTAGE - PRO – CHART V

LOWER BODY EXERCISES [Mon., Wed., Fri.]
[Use light resistance bands for Exercises 2, 3, 4, 5]

1 - Warm up	2 - Hamstring Blasts	3 - Lunges
4 - Calf Extensions	5 - Squats	6 - Run

PROGRESS SCHEDULE – Lower Body Chart V

Date	Weight	Level	1	2	3	4	5	6
		1	3 min.	21	11	16	31	410
		2	3 min.	22	11	17	32	420
		3	3 min.	23	12	18	33	430
		4	3 min.	24	12	19	34	440
		5	3 min.	25	13	20	35	450
		6	3 min.	26	13	21	36	460
		7	3 min.	27	14	22	37	470
		8	3 min.	28	14	23	38	480
		9	3 min.	29	15	24	39	490
		10	3 min.	30	15	25	40	500

UPPER BODY EXERCISES [Tues., Thurs., Sat.]
[Use medium resistance bands for Exercises 10, 11, 13, 14 15, 16]

1 - Warm up	7 - Bird Dog		8 - Side Bridge	9 - Curl-Up
10 - Tricep Extension	11 - Upright Rowing	12 - Chair Dips	13 - Bicep Curls	14 - Chest Press
15 - Lawn Mower		16 - Forearm Blasts		17 - Pushups

PROGRESS SCHEDULE – Upper Body Chart V

	1	7	8	9	10	11	12	13	14	15	16	17
4	3 min.	2	2	16	11	11	16	6	16	11	16	11
2	3 min.	2	2	16	11	12	17	6	17	12	17	11
3	3 min.	2	2	17	12	13	18	7	18	13	18	12
4	3 min.	2	2	17	12	14	19	7	19	14	19	12
5	3 min.	2	2	18	13	15	20	8	20	15	20	13
6	3 min.	2	2	18	13	16	21	8	21	16	21	13
7	3 min.	2	2	19	14	17	22	9	22	17	22	14
8	3 min.	2	2	19	14	18	23	9	23	18	23	14
9	3 min.	2	2	20	15	19	24	10	24	19	24	15
10	3 min.	2	2	20	15	20	25	10	25	20	25	15

EXERCISE ADVANTAGE - PRO – CHART VI

LOWER BODY EXERCISES [Mon., Wed., Fri.]
[Use medium resistance band for Exercises 2, 3, 4, 5]

1 - Warm up	2 - Hamstring Blasts	3 - Lunges
4 - Calf Extensions	5 - Squats	6 - Run

PROGRESS SCHEDULE – Lower Body Chart VI

Date	Weight	Level	1	2	3	4	5	6
		1	3 min.	21	11	16	31	410
		2	3 min.	22	11	17	32	420
		3	3 min.	23	12	18	33	430
		4	3 min.	24	12	19	34	440
		5	3 min.	25	13	20	35	450
		6	3 min.	26	13	21	36	460
		7	3 min.	27	14	22	37	470
		8	3 min.	28	14	23	38	480
		9	3 min.	29	15	24	39	490
		10	3 min.	30	15	25	40	500

UPPER BODY EXERCISES [Tues., Thurs., Sat.]
Use heavy resistance band for Exercises 10, 11, 13, 14 15, 16

1 - Warm up	7 - Bird Dog	8 - Side Bridge	9 - Curl-Up	
10 - Tricep Extension	11 - Upright Rowing	12 - Chair Dips	13 - Bicep Curls	14 - Chest Press
15 - Lawn Mower		16 - Forearm Blasts	17 - Pushups	

PROGRESS SCHEDULE – Upper Body Chart VI

	1	7	8	9	10	11	12	13	14	15	16	17
1	3 min.	2	3	11	11	11	21	6	16	11	16	16
2	3 min.	2	3	11	11	12	22	6	17	12	17	16
3	3 min.	2	3	12	12	13	23	7	18	13	18	17
4	3 min.	2	3	12	12	14	24	7	19	14	19	17
5	3 min.	2	3	13	13	15	25	8	20	15	20	18
6	3 min.	2	3	13	13	16	26	8	21	16	21	18
7	3 min.	2	3	14	14	17	27	9	22	17	22	19
8	3 min.	2	3	14	14	18	28	9	23	18	23	19
9	3 min.	2	3	15	15	19	29	10	24	19	24	20
10	3 min.	2	3	15	15	20	30	10	25	20	25	20

EXERCISE ADVANTAGE - PRO – CHART VII

LOWER BODY EXERCISES [Mon., Wed., Fri.]
Use heavy resistance bands for Exercises 2, 3, 4, 5

1 - Warm up	2 - Hamstring Blasts	3 - Lunges
4 - Calf Extensions	5 - Squats	6 - Run

PROGRESS SCHEDULE – Lower Body Chart VII

Date	Weight	Level	1	2	3	4	5	6
		1	3 min.	21	11	16	31	410
		2	3 min.	22	11	17	32	420
		3	3 min.	23	12	18	33	430
		4	3 min.	24	12	19	34	440
		5	3 min.	25	13	20	35	450
		6	3 min.	26	13	21	36	460
		7	3 min.	27	14	22	37	470
		8	3 min.	28	14	23	38	480
		9	3 min.	29	15	24	39	490
		10	3 min.	30	15	25	40	500

UPPER BODY EXERCISES [Tues., Thurs., Sat.]
Use heavy resistance band for Exercises 10, 11, 13, 14 15, 16

1 - Warm up	7 - Bird Dog	8 - Side Bridge	9 - Curl-Up
10 - Tricep Extension	11 - Upright Rowing	12 - Chair Dips	13 - Bicep Curls	14 - Chest Press
15 - Lawn Mower	16 - Forearm Blasts	17 - Pushups

PROGRESS SCHEDULE – Upper Body Chart VII

	1	7	8	9	10	11	12	13	14	15	16	17
1	3 min.	2	3	16	16	21	26	11	26	21	26	21
2	3 min.	2	3	16	16	21	27	11	26	21	26	21
3	3 min.	2	3	17	17	22	28	12	27	22	27	22
4	3 min.	2	3	17	17	22	29	12	27	22	27	22
5	3 min.	2	3	18	18	23	30	13	28	23	28	23
6	3 min.	2	3	18	18	23	31	13	28	23	28	23
7	3 min.	2	3	19	19	24	32	14	29	24	29	24
8	3 min.	2	3	19	19	24	33	14	28	24	29	24
9	3 min.	2	3	20	20	25	34	15	30	25	30	25
10	3 min.	2	3	20	20	25	35	15	30	25	30	25

EXERCISE DESCRIPTIONS

Resistance bands are required, and it is recommended that men obtain bands in weights of 20, 40, and 50 pounds, and women and children a size lighter in each. Resistance can be modified by where the bands are gripped. It will take a little time, effort, and practice to work into these exercises, but muscle-memory will quickly be developed.

1 - Warmup

Lower Body Exercise: Walk in place one minute. Pump elbows down when either knee goes up, and pump arms upward as feet touch down. Do stretches 4–8.
Upper Body Exercise: Same, except do stretches 1-4.

2 - Hamstring Blasts

1. On hands and knees, Place resistance band around one foot and hold ends in each hand, ends taut.
2. Extend leg straight back, squeezing glutes. Return to start position.
3. Do total reps, then repeat with other leg.

3 - Lunges

1. Standing, step back on one foot approximately 2 feet. Place band under front foot and hold ends in each hand, ends stretched. Keep head and back erect, in a neutral position.
2. Lower body by bending at hips and knees until thigh is parallel to floor. Return to start position.
3. Do total reps, then repeat with other leg.

4 - Calf Extensions

1. Standing erect, step on band with one foot near handle. Hold other end, stretched. Lift other foot.
2. Do up and down [tiptoe] movement on one foot, holding in tiptoe position for 1 sec.
3. Do total reps, then repeat with other leg.

5 - Squats

1. Standing, feet shoulder width apart. Step on the middle of the band, holding at shoulder level with each hand, stretched tight (i.e. contracted position for bicep curl).
2. Slowly do a full squat [knees at 90°], hold one second, return to the starting position.

6 - Run

Chart IV: Run in place. Do 20 "fast feet" *and* 20 jumping jacks each 100 paces, or run 1 mile in 8 minutes.
Chart V: Same, except "high knee" running, hands on head, last *full* 100 paces, or run 1 mile in 7 minutes.
Chart VI: Same, except "high knee" running, hands on head, last two *full*

sets of 100 paces, or run 1 mile in 6 minutes.

Chart VII: Same, except "high knee" running, hands on head, last three *full* sets of 100 paces, or run 1 mile in 5½ minutes.

7 - Bird Dog
1. On hands and knees, stiffen and hold abs, then extend one arm and the opposite leg.
2. Stretch and hold 2 reps of 15 seconds each.
3. Repeat other side.

8 - Side Bridge
Chart IV: 1. Lie on side, propped up on forearm. Tighten abs. Raise hips, with feet, hips, and shoulders locked in a straight line. Hold 15 sec., then roll on forearms to other side and repeat. Do 2 reps each side.
Chart V: 2 reps of 20 sec. for each side.
Chart VI: 3 reps of 15 sec. for each side.
Chart VII: 3 reps of 20 sec. for each side.

9 - Curlup
Chart IV: Lie on back, one knee bent, hands under lumbar. Stiffen abs, then lift head and back off floor, together from the breastbone. Do not poke chin forward or rest shoulders on ground. Hold 5 sec.
Chart V: Same.
Chart VI: Same, except elbows off floor at all times.
Chart VII: Same

10 - Tricep Extension
1. Stand, one foot in front, and step on one band handle with rear foot. Hold band taut behind head.
2. Extend hand upward until arm is fully extended.
3. Do total reps, then repeat with other arm.

11 - Upright Rowing
1. Stand with one foot in front, on middle of band, hands together at waist, holding ends of band in hands.
2. Pull the band upward with both hands, supple wrists, to the chin, with hands close to the body. Elbows extend out, ending above ears.

12 - Chair Dips
Chart IV: Men: hands 6 inches out from shoulders; knees bent. Women: hands 6 inches out from shoulders; knees bent; legs in scissor position.
Chart V: Men: hands under shoulders; knees bent. Women: Same as men on Chart IV.
Chart VI: Men: hands out 6 inches; straight legs. Women: Same as men on Chart V.

Chart VII: Men: Hands under shoulders; straight legs. Women: Same as men VI.

13 - Bicep Curls
1. Stand, one foot slightly back on middle of band. Arms at sides, grasping each end of band and holding taut, with both hands in underhand grip (palms facing forward), and elbows close to sides.
2. Flex at the elbows and curl the band up to approximately shoulder level. Keep elbows close to sides.
3. Do total reps in each of 3 different motions: Wide (curl with wrists out 6 inches from shoulders); Regular (curl with wrists straight ahead); Cross (alternate arms; hands crossing chest). Upper arms do not move.

14 - Chest Press
1. Lie on back with band under back, holding one band handle in one hand and the band in the other. Pull band across the chest, stretching it as tight as possible.
2. Press fist with handle up toward ceiling, and return to starting position.
3. Do total reps, then repeat with other arm.

15 - Lawn Mower
1. Stand with left leg in front and right leg behind, with handle of band in right hand, palm facing inward and band taut under left foot, left forearm resting on left thigh.
2. With back straight, body leaning forward, pull band toward body as if starting a lawn mower.
3. Do total reps, then repeat on other side.

16 - Forearm Blasts
1. Sit in chair, feet on middle of band, arms on thighs, palms down, holding band in each hand.
2. Curl wrists up to shoulders and down in slow, intentional movement. Hold in the up position for ½ sec.
3. Do total reps, then repeat with palms facing up.

17 - Pushups
Push-ups [varying hand locations]: Narrow [inside shoulders], Regular [under shoulders], Wide [outside shoulders]. Do total number of reps each way, except wide to failure.

Section Three - OUTLINES

To my Children:

The Greeks were perhaps first to realize the inevitable connection between a healthy mind and a healthy body. A happy, successful life requires both, and more and more studies are proving the magnitude of that connection. Even susceptibility to disease is largely determined by emotional health and, since humans are inevitably social animals, by the ability to get along well with others, particularly family.

Despite extreme cynicism toward the educational system, I have the highest regard for education. Among thousands of books read, there have been some that seemed to be of particular import. When I read, I sideline the important things, and then go back and read the sidelines. If I believe a book is really important, I then write an outline from the sidelines, which takes only a few hours. The outline can then be referred to on a continuing basis.

Several books dealing with physical and mental health have seemed paramount. To help you, perhaps, better understand these books, I am providing you with the outlines of a few of them. My approach to education is to study only things I really want to understand. Memory only comes with motivation. So think about why these outlines can be important to you, read just the ones that are interesting, and think about the concepts.

I can't save you from the aches and pains of life—but I would surely like to save you from the stupid mistakes I have made! I wish you good health, happiness, and success.

Dad

THE CHINA STUDY

T Colin Campbell PhD

INTRODUCTION

America's health is failing: 2/3 are overweight, 15 million have diabetes, 100
  million have high cholesterol, the war against heart disease and cancer is
  being lost, young people increasingly are contracting "adult" diseases.
Dr Campbell spent 40 years studying diet at the most advanced research levels
  [He grew up on a farm, and began research for the beef industry, but changed
his position when his father died from heart disease caused by too much meat.]
  Genes are implicated, but do not cause diseases: they predispose contracting
them
  Animal proteins in the bloodstream are the common trigger
  Good diet is the single most powerful weapon against disease
  Live longer and healthier, arrest and reverse disease, look younger and
    have more energy, lose weight, increase mental acuity, avoid doctors.
    The price: Eat right
Heart disease, diabetes, obesity, cancer, autoimmune diseases, etc. can often
be *reversed*
  People who eat the *least* animal protein, and the most natural plants, get the
least disease
  Plants need to be in their whole, unrefined state
  People who eat the *most* animal protein [the "American" diet] get the most
disease
  Dairy foods, particularly cow's milk, greatly increase risk of disease
  Atkins and South Beach diets are deadly: Sacrifice long-term health to
short-term loss

DISEASES OF AFFLUENCE

Compared to less "advanced" cultures, Americans are dying from diseases of
affluence
  Heart disease, cancer, diabetes, stroke, alzheimers, obesity, MS,
osteoporosis, etc
  The same diet that is good for one of these is good for all the others
If a vegetarian diet seems "impractical", how "practical" is obesity, disease,
surgery, etc?
Heart disease
  In one study, 77% of Americans in their *20s* had serious signs of incipient
heart disease
  A test was made of 18 people who had suffered, collectively, 49 serious
coronary "events"
    They were all put on a plant-based diet, with no drugs
    In 11 years there was only 1 event, an angina attack—from a patient who

stopped the diet

[By comparison, American medicine's solution is to recommend ½ an aspirin a day]

Obesity

2/3 of American adults are overweight; half of those are obese—and it's growing [a pun]

The first thing visitors from other countries notice is how heavy Americans are

Permanent weight loss results from a whole food, plant-based diet, with reasonable exercise

People who eat all they want lose 10-17 lbs in 3 weeks

Diabetes [costs America $130 billion each year]

Diabetics are subject to getting all the other "affluent diseases", as well as many others

Type 1 [5 – 10% of diabetics] begins in childhood or adolescence

Body cannot produce insulin because pancreas destroyed

An autoimmune disease that has been linked to infant feeding of cow's milk

Genes predispose, but casein is the "trigger". Slowly-decreasing danger continues to age 14

Type 2 used to be called "adult onset", but is occurring in younger and younger people

Pancreas produces insulin, but it doesn't do its job. Often results from obesity

Diet is crucial to diabetics: Reduce animal proteins and increase whole, unrefined plant food

Deaths from diabetes are reduced by this diet from 20.4/100,000 to 2.9/100,000

After 3 weeks on a vegetarian diet, Type 1 diabetics lowered insulin medication up to 40%

Most Type 2 diabetics can stop insulin entirely [24 of 25 in one study]

Cancer

All studies show more cancer in societies eating more animal protein

Many chemicals are carcinogens, but they usually act as a trigger only from animal proteins

In lab tests, rats were fed aflatoxin, a cancer-causing chemical

Rats who had 20% protein, from cow's milk, *all* got cancer; if 5% protein, *none* did

20% animal protein is what Americans consume as a typical diet

In the test, cancer could be turned on/off, by feeding/witholding animal protein!

All forms of cancer are subject to the same effects of diet, both pro and con

E.g., Breast cancer is linked to high levels of female hormones, increased by animal protein

Genes only predispose the disease, not determine it. A plant-based diet counters the causes

[Note: a recent study showed vitamin D can arrest, and even reverse, cancer]

Autoimmune Diseases

Includes Hyper/hypo-thyroid, MS, arthritis, lupus, type 1 diabetes, Crohn's disease, etc.

250,000 Americans newly diagnosed each year

The body attacks itself, often triggered by a virus

More prevalent farther from equator, with use of cow's milk and less Vitamin D

If caught in early stages can be reversed; can be slowed if caught later

When this book was written, 18 of 19 people on the National Academy of Science's Food and Nutrition Board represented the meat, dairy, and egg industries

They label research about diseases and causes "controversial" to keep them from the public

Similar to how the connection between smoking and lung cancer was obfuscated for years

They spend $100s of millions each year to thwart findings they don't like

They control the recommendations of the Academy, which are adopted by our Government:

Recommend up to 35% of calories from protein [no other authority recommends more than 10%], up to 35% from fat, up to 65% from carbs, and up to 25% from refined sugar!

Based on their "findings" the following is an adequate diet:

Breakfast: Fruitloops with skim milk, package of M&Ms, fiber and vitamin supplements.

Lunch: Cheeseburger. Dinner: 3 slices pepperoni pizza, 16 oz. soda, sugar cookies

These standards are used for all Government-financed programs, including school lunches

GOOD NUTRITION PRINCIPLES:

Nutrition is the combined activities of many foods, in complex chemical interactions

The whole is greater than the sum of the parts. Supplements cannot substitute for good diet

Vitamins D and B12 are the only supplements recommended. Do not overdose on D

There are no animal nutrients that are not better provided by plants

Genes do not determine disease on their own. Nutrition determines whether they are activated

Good nutrition, to a large extent, can control the effects of noxious chemicals

The same nutrition that prevents disease can stop or even reverse it

The same nutrition good for one disease is generally good for all others

Eat all you want of whole, unrefined plant foods [precluding white flour, refined sugar, etc]

Eat only a minimum of other foods, but don't obsess about it

Even after a month you will feel better, and begin to lose weight

CHANGE YOUR BRAIN, CHANGE YOUR LIFE
-Daniel Amen, M.D., PhD [PBS Program]

SPECT brain scans of healthy and unhealthy brains [using radioactive
    isotopes]:
  Unhealthy brains looked like swiss cheese—"holes" for all the dead sections
  Factors that contribute: Genetics, brain injury, heart disease, illegal drugs,
    lack of physical and brain exercise, overweight, diabetes, depression,
    A.D.H.D., cancer treatment, sleep apnea, cosmetics
  Most damage is from drugs, alcohol, caffeine, smoking, toxic fumes
Now know brain cells can be partly regenerated with proper treatment
Three sections of the brain:
  1. Prefrontal Cortex: ["Executive"]. [30% of human brain; small in animals]
    The part that makes us human: Forethought, impulse control, maturity,
      empathy, cooperation
    If not functioning properly [underactive]: Poor judgment, short attention
      span, A.D.H.D., weak conscience, lack of persistence, thrill junkie
    To fix: Write out goals and read them daily, exercise 4 times weekly, eat
      high protein low carb diet, take fish oil
  2. Cingulate section: ["Gear shifter"]
    Changes focus, encourages cooperation, sees options, detects errors
    If not functioning properly [overactive]: O.C.D., hold grudges,
      argumentative, perfectionist, rigid, micromanage
    To fix: Increase Seratonin, get up and move to distract yourself,
      consciously set up options, exercise, high carb low, protein diet
  3. Limbic section: [Emotion]
    Processes happiness, pain, moods, libido, bonding
    If not functioning properly: Depression, bipolar, negative attitude, low self
      esteem, anger, guilt, low libido, ANTS [automatic negative thoughts]
      "Anteaters": Challenge negative thoughts - argue with yourself, each
        day write 5 things you're grateful for, exercise [better than drugs for
        clinical depression], take fish oil
Rules to Improve Brain, reduce brain loss, and encourage growth of new cells
  Protect your brain physically: Avoid potential injury, get enough sleep,
    avoid brain toxins [alcohol, caffeine, toxic fumes, cosmetics]
  Eat brain foods: Lean protein, salmon, tuna, turkey, complex carbs,
    vegetables, lots of water, blueberries, broccoli, decaf green tea, oatmeal,
    oranges, spinach, walnuts, vitamins, iron
  Exercise your brain: Learn every day - work it hard at *new* things for 15
    minutes
  Exercise your body: Aerobic exercise that requires coordination and results
    in heavy sweating

Coordination exercises the brain; sweating rids the body of toxins

Normal to lose 85,000 brain cells per day as one ages

Early signs of: Alzheimer's: Difficulty smelling strawberries, pineapple, lemons, natural gas

Alzheimer's can be reversed if caught in very early stages

To fix: Avoid brain toxins, exercise body 4 times weekly and brain every day, eat brain foods, sleep enough and well

THE POWER OF OPTIMISM

--McGinnis

If you follow the following principles, you will always be mentally healthy and functional, and you will never need a psychologist.

"TOUGH-MINDED OPTIMISM"
Realistic acceptance of reality, combined with hope
As effective as psychotherapy, if no major depression
Pessimism leads to cynicism: no faith so no effort
Comparison with other self-help philosophies:
  "Power of positive thinking" implies no limits, which
      is unrealistic
    "Everything will turn out fine" encourages passivity and
fatalism
    "You create your own reality" is crap
    "My family was dysfunctional" abrogates responsibility
ANTICIPATE PROBLEMS
Accept and verbalize them--pain is part of life
Look for the good in bad situations, but not phony pep talks
Use bad for a good lesson--look for and accept the lesson
Don't be Pollyanna--much is impossible
Be a problem solver--try to make at least some difference
Look for options, even though none is excellent
Get started--it's half the battle
ACCEPT PARTIAL SOLUTIONS
Don't be a perfectionist--be flexible
Accept what cannot be changed; give up if necessary
Try a lot; have many failures, but many successes
You won't find life worth living; make it worth living
Half of something is better than all of nothing
BELIEVE YOU CONTROL YOUR FUTURE
Do something initially to generate small successes
Face reality as it is; change yourself if necessary
Exercise will; choose your attitude
Believe you have almost unlimited capacity
Believe your best is yet to be
INCREASE YOUR ENERGY
Entropy: all systems run down--must reenergize
Associate with energetic people, including children
Expand interests and knowledge--try new things
Develop spiritually--use the Sabbath

INTERRUPT NEGATIVE THOUGHTS
Monitor thoughts--negative ones are a habit
Displace them with good thoughts
Snap a rubber band on your wrist for each bad thought
Try to view things in a more favorable light
Choose not to be defensive
You can't choose how you feel--but you *can* choose how you react

PRACTICE ADMIRATION AND GRATITUDE
Say "thank you"; admire things which are good
Be grateful; enjoy what you have

REHEARSE SUCCESS
Think in. pictures; it's even more effective than practice
Imagination is more important than knowledge
Avoid worry and develop faith
Complaining is a habit; don't rehearse failure
Always talk about the good news--concentrate on successes

PRACTICE LOVE
Serve others and have a basic belief in human nature
Avoid hostility by tolerance and forgiveness

Do these things!
Even if you don't understand it, do these things!
Even if you don't *feel* like it, *do these things!*

HAPPINESS

"Happiness is the design and object of our existence, and will be the end thereof if we pursue the path that leads to it." –Joseph Smith

"People are about as happy as they make up their mind to be." –Abraham Lincoln

"People worry a lot about happiness. If they'd quit worrying about it and get on with doing what they need to be doing, they'd be a whole lot less unhappy". –RC

20/20 News Program, January 2008

Determinants of Happiness

1. 50% is in the genes, e.g. some people just seem to be "born happy"
2. 10% is circumstances, e.g. childhood, looks, health, status, where live
3. 40% is intentional attitudes and choices, particularly:
   Goals and their pursuit
   Relationships, with the ability and effort to develop and maintain them
   Positive meditation: Kind thoughts, compassion, counting blessings
      Half hour each day can make the change in 2 weeks!

Fundamentals of Happiness

1. Certain things create feelings of happiness, e.g. socializing, praying, sex
   Happiness is not a "state"; it comes in moments of time
   Having kids was not shown necessarily to give happiness
2. Money: Have enough [a little more than friends], and spend it well
3. All happiness has a social basis: Not what you do, but who you do it with
   The happiest people have a rich social life
4. Have a life "calling", or use sheer will to turn your work into one
5. Develop "flow". Easy to do with something you love; follow your bliss

Happiest places on earth [US is 23rd]

Denmark is the happiest country
   Despite 63% tax rate and, paradoxically, a high suicide rate
   A homogeneous society: 9 of 10 are full-blood Danes, 8 of 10 Lutheran
      All jobs have similar pay and status, and strong trust of each other
      Everyone is well provided for; few rich and little desire for it
      As Muslims, and conflict, increase in population, happiness is declining
   92% of Danes belong to one or more government-sponsored social clubs
Singapore has the happiest people in Asia
   Again, paradoxically, with a high suicide rate
   Happiness despite extremely strict laws and high taxes
      E.g. beaten with a cane for spitting in public
      They believe US has too much freedom!
   The country is clean, safe, stable, and economically secure

Corruption is discouraged by paying top gov't officials $1mm per year
They are more materialistic than the Danes, and somewhat less content
The few rich people feel least secure, and want even more
Unhappiest places have extreme poverty, instability, or insecurity
E. g. starving countries in Africa
Italians are least happy in Europe, because of total corruption

The Effects of Success on Happiness -ABC News program, circa 1992
Americans who were interviewed expressed several expectations:
Most believe money is the key
But studies proved newly rich are only happy for about a year
Then, no matter how much they have, it is not enough and they want more
Many spend compulsively to maintain "happiness", till bankrupt
Those who seek fame, as expected, are happy only as long as it continues
The ambitious are happy only as long as they continue to climb upward
Must continue to exceed the apparent success of others
Conclusion: All these things fail to bring real or lasting happiness
Contrary to these beliefs, several principles are conducive to real happiness:
Need to believe we have substantial control in our life
Found even among babies a few months old
Most important factor, ahead of money, for employees
Feel in control only if accept responsibility for things that happen to you
Need to be optimistic: Believe you can deal with inevitable problems
With optimism, defeat spurs you on, rather than beating you down
Need to work. Leisure is a curse to happiness
Need to experience challenge and the opportunity for achievement
While working in pursuit of other things, happiness happens
Need to have close relationships to which we are committed
Relationships, e.g. marriage, often break up when success occurs
Unhappiness follows
Need to believe something is more important than ourselves
Faith in God, and service to him, is a usual underpinning to happiness
Gives sense of purpose and of commitment to something greater

Miscellany
The top 10 happiest states and their well-being scores (out of a possible 100 points):

Utah: 69.2	Minnesota: 67.3	California: 67
Hawaii: 68.2	Maryland: 67.1	Arizona: 66.8
Wyoming: 68	Washington: 67.1	
Colorado: 67.3	Massachusetts: 67	

Jean Chatsky, "Money" Magazine, polled 1,500 people
Annual income over $50,000 makes no difference to happiness
Simmons and Chatsky: Work, religion, and family make people happy
Dr John Izzo, who studies happiness, interviewed 250 people age 60-106.
They *all* agreed there are five true secrets to happiness: Be true to self,
Leave no regrets, Become love, Live the moment, Give more than you take.
Suicide rates/100,000: Russia: 34.3. Japan: 24. Denmark: 13.6. Sweden: 13.2.
Iceland: 12.6. Canada: 11.9. Norway: 11.5. U.S: 11. Singapore: 9.5. Italy: 7.1.
U.K: 7. Jamaica: 0.1.

Conclusions
- Achieving happiness can be accomplished, and is therefore worth the effort!
  Circumstances [10%] can be worked on to a degree
    Attitude and activities [40%] can be worked on a lot
- Look for something greater than self
    E.g. God, a cause, community, service, etc
- Many have negative mental tapes that say, "I'm not happy, shouldn't be
  happy, don't deserve to be happy". Those tapes need to be fought
    Spend time daily reading "feel-good" stories to displace negative tapes
- Maintain many good social contacts and close relationships, e.g. family
- Have short- and long-term goals. Work on career, hobbies, travel, etc
- Avoid materialism, but work on having enough to comfortably meet needs
- Deal with and resolve the problems in your life

THIS IS A TERRIBLE WORLD, FILLED WITH VIOLENCE AND HATE
THIS IS A WONDERFUL WORLD, FILLED WITH KINDNESS AND LOVE
WHICH WORLD DO YOU CHOOSE TO SEE?
WHICH WORLD DO YOU CHOOSE TO LIVE IN?   -RC

THE 7 HABITS OF HIGHLY EFFECTIVE PEOPLE

--Stephen R. Covey

Even many who have great outward success feel like--and are--failures. It shows in their relationships with themselves and with others. They are deeply unhappy, even as they seem to enjoy success. During the past 50 years there has been an emphasis on the "personality ethic": public image, social consciousness, techniques for success, quick fixes. Prior to that the emphasis was on a "character ethic": integrity, courage, justice, patience, hard work, and the golden rule. The former focuses on the development of skills, the latter on the development of character. The former is manipulative, the latter tries to build others as well as oneself. The character ethic requires internalization of the following habits, developed through desire, knowledge, and continual practice. The goal is to grow from dependence, through independence, toward a synergistic interdependence.

Private Victory
  1] **Be proactive**: You are responsible. *Choose* your responses
    To the actions of others and to events that occur
  2] **Begin with the end in mind**: This is a "spiritual creation"
    Set specific goals and specific plans to achieve them
  3] **Put first things first**: This is a principle of pragmatic faith
    Get to work and do things in order

Public Victory
  4] **Think win/win**: If everyone involved does not win, it is not worth doing
  5] **Seek first to understand, then to be understood**: Have you ever noticed in arguments people do not even listen to the other side?
  6] **Synergize**: Move through dependence to independence to interdependence. Think what little you could accomplish if you had to do everything yourself!

Renewal
  7] **Sharpen the saw**: Education, recreation, spiritual renewal, friends, exercise. All things in balance

LIFE STRATEGIES

-- Phil McGraw

1: You either "get it" or you don't. Be honest with yourself.
2: You create your own experience. Take responsibility.
3: People do what works. Look for the payoffs, for self, others.
4: You can't change what you won't admit. Face reality.
5: Life rewards action. [Ready, fire, aim!]
6: There is no reality, only perception. [A⇒B⇒C. Not A⇒C].
7: Life is managed, it is not cured. Take charge of it.
8: You teach people how to treat you. Look at payoffs.
9: If you don't forgive, it will destroy you.
10: You have to name it to claim it. What do you want?

Get Real
The world is highly competitive and there ain't no Santa Claus
　There's no point whining about it
What is needed is a clear, knowledge-based strategy
　To overcome problems and fulfill goals
Society is a disaster, and people are not trained to manage their lives
　No one is taught how to be married, a parent, to manage their life, etc
　There are idiots with degrees who don't know how to get out of the rain
　For a successful life, you must have a life strategy
Most are in denial about their problems
　Are you sick enough of your life to be willing to change?
　Most are afraid to test, or even recognize their assumptions
　　They just want them to be true
Problems do not resolve themselves
　Inertia: you have to be willing to change, and make an initial effort
　Indicators: Frustrated, in a rut, bored, just hanging on, in a comfort zone, failing, lonely, depressed
Don't just need insight—need to change right now
　Assignment 1: List the top 5 things you have failed to fully admit to yourself about yourself
　Look for poor life-management skills
　Assignment 2: Write "The Story I'll Tell Myself If I don't Make Meaningful Change"
　Where will you be? Why? What will you rationalize?
　Have to accomplish 3 things: Learn yourself thoroughly and honestly; Learn the real ways of the world; Learn a life strategy to set and obtain goals

Life Law 1: You either get it or you don't
If don't get it you will fail, and live in great pain

You have to know how the world works
You have to find what makes you and others tick, to get self and others to do what you want, connect with others, and predict outcomes
You have to have knowledge and skills necessary to create the results you want

If you don't, you'd better get used to being a have-not

Assignment 3: Look at the patterns of things you do in all areas of your life. Make a list of everything you take on blind faith that does not work

Maya Angelou: "You did what you knew how to do, and when you knew better you did better"

Understanding someone: What do they value? Want? Experiences and beliefs? Fears and prejudices? Common grounds? Feelings about self?
Greatest fear is rejection; greatest need is acceptance

Must protect self esteem. Get what they want; talk about what they want.

Respond only to what they understand.

Are often petty. Have hidden agendas. Wear a mask
Most imp person to influence: you

Need to enhance positive characteristics, eliminate negative

Need to influence others so they feel good around you and know will be lifted up and motivated

LL 2: You create your own experience
Acknowledge and accept accountability for your life. Fault is not relevant—do not assign fault, to yourself or anyone else

Overcome perfectionism and judgments

Give yourself permission to be less than perfect, and to have accumulated baggage

People who fail always have someone else to blame

Finding fault creates a negative physiology, and programs failure
Whatever attitudes, relations, job satisfaction, health, you are accountable

If do not believe this, then accepting that you have no control. You are a passive victim

If don't believe this, then will misdiagnose every problem and event in your life

Recognize that everything is a choice and you are the result of your choices

Recognize the rule of reciprocity: you get what you give

Examine the style you have in dealing with people, and recognize how that affects their response

List the rough edges, and work at eliminating them
If believe you are right about non-accountability you can and will do nothing to change it

If people won't listen, it is your responsibility they do not understand you

Whatever situation, must believe the solution is within you

Must stop saying, "Why are they doing this to me", and say, "Why doing this to myself". "What thoughts, communications, behaviors can I change to change the result"

Assignment 4: List the 5 most significant times in life when you were a victim. Describe in enough detail to capture the emotion of it. Determine how you contributed substantially to the result

Assignment 5: Make a written list of your top 10 negative tapes. Carry a card, and list each as it comes up. Stop the tapes!

LL 3: People do what works
You have to identify the payoffs that drive your behavior and that of others. They have to be there

Control the payoffs to control your life. Have to control the cause and effect relationship

Payoffs are addictive, especially if they allow you to avoid pain

The real payoff may be very difficult to identify. Some are extremely unhealthy, some are good

Often we do things *knowing* that it will not be for our best. Recognize that at some level they work

Cannot eliminate negative behavior without knowing why it is done. To "get it" have to know

The payoff may be unconscious, even though we consciously know it is negative

Must look for the unconscious and conscious payoffs, and relative strength

E.g. parents may teach a child to scream and demand by rewarding that behavior by responding

Examine your relationships and determine what negative behavior you are rewarding

Look for the negative payoffs in your own life. Must stop paying yourself for negative behavior

When you sabotage yourself, there is a payoff. Must find and break it to stop the vicious circle

Often when found the power disappears

Assignment 6: Describe in detail the 5 most frustrating and negative behaviors in your life. Analyze the payoff you are getting from each, how your needs are "met". May be acceptance, rejection, fear, avoiding risk or work, immediate vs. delayed gratification

LL 4: You can't change what you don't acknowledge
You have to be truthful and stop making excuses about what is not working in your life

Most do not want truth, they want validation—reinforcement whether right or wrong

People want to be right more than anything else

If you won't take ownership of your role and responsibility you can do nothing

Bad habits become more and more entrenched

Have to be honest about where you are right now or will destroy your whole strategy for life

Lies come either by misrepresentation or by omission. They can even kill you

We lie to ourselves unconsciously, through denial, so have to make a real effort

Must look for and analyze warning signs in attitudes, behavior, and results

Need to look at every area that is not working in life. Must be absolutely brutal

If don't do this, we are cheating ourselves. Doing so is our first positive step

If admit a problem, and responsibility for it, living with it becomes very difficult. You're half there

Acknowledge: your problem, need knowledge, getting a payoff, personal characteristics leading to failure. If this causes pain that is a good thing—it will motivate change. Use it to advantage!

It's difficult to make meaningful substantial changes. You cannot do it without total honesty

LL 5: Life rewards action

Make careful decisions, then pull the trigger. No one cares about intentions, they just look at results

The only thing that matters is action and results. It is the only way to measure yourself

When you choose the action you choose the consequence. It needs to be purposeful and directed

Assignment 7: Are you in a rut? List and examine your recurring activities

Do you make promises to yourself and others and not keep them? Do you let others do that?

Procrastination: Ever moment you fail to act is another moment wasted. If not now, when?

BE committed, DO what is necessary, HAVE what you want

Knowledge, insights, and understanding must be translated into action

The difference between winners and losers is winners do the things losers won't do

Faith without works is dead. If you don't have it's because you don't act

Begin, and new possibilities will come. Be willing to risk, and persist

Assignment 8: Make a list of the 5-10 most important people. Write down for each what would be left unsaid if one of you died now

Assignment 9: List the top priorities in each of the following categories:

Personal	Relational	Professional	Familial	Spiritual

LL 6: There is no reality, only perception

You need to identify the filters through which you see the world

Those with really bizarre filters are insane

No matter what happens to you, how you interpret it is entirely your choice. You give it meaning and value. Choose the one leading to your goals

Recognize the perception other people are placing—and that there is invariably a difference

Perception is not that something bad is good, fair or unfair, but that you can deal with it

Conclusion you draw from your filter is either you can or cannot deal with it

The cards you are dealt in life are what they are. All that matters is how you play them

If you choose to look through the filter of the past you cannot deal with the present

You may be allowing an event in the past to control and destroy your life now

Identify and analyze the filters, e.g. prejudices, that are controlling your present life

Your strategy may be entirely correct, but if your filter is wrong it will fail

You have to test your operating assumptions before relying on them

The filters through which we view ourselves are the least accurate

May fail to recognize negatives, particularly our own accountability

Undoubtedly fail to give credit for qualities and abilities

Look for yourself in the mirror held up by others, but pick the right mirrors!

Keep an open mind about yourself—our perceptions create our limiting beliefs

Like the elephant at the stake, we cannot go beyond them

If you can control your perceptions, you can control your interpretations and attitudes

That is power

You need to really shake up your belief system. Challenge all your views about yourself

The world, and you, can look completely new

Assignment 10: Search for your limiting beliefs. You have to really dig: they are really imperceptible and insidious. They probably go way back. Your "tapes" are examples

LL 7: Life is managed, it is not cured

Learn to take charge of your life and hang on. Think of yourself as the manager of your life

Is he doing a good job, or do you need to get after him?

Is he doing a good job for the others for whom there is responsibility?

Job Description: Acknowledge the life laws apply to you; commit to resolve rather than endure problems; face the "what-if" questions and answer them, e.g. "What if I get fired?"; refuse to live with unfinished emotional business, causing overreactions to small issues; honor your agreements with self and others

Life has momentum and direction. Take conscious responsibility for those

Define wants in terms of goals and give them project status. Create a To-do list and priorities

Assignment 11: Write down all your conscious life decisions. What do you demand of yourself; What are you willing to accept from yourself? Looking at your actions, are you living in a comfort zone? Make a decision to ramp up, and consider each day how to do that

Consider for each area of your life. Apply the laws of life to each

We need to try to make the right decisions, but sometimes we need to make a decision right

Poor choices test maturity and resolve

LL 8: We teach people how to treat us

Accept responsibility for, rather than complain about, how people treat you

Have a right to be treated with fairness and respect, but must teach people to do it

Be sure, by reviewing the life laws, you're not at fault—the principle of reciprocity

Relationships are mutually defined, by an intrinsic negotiation in the relationship

In therapy for couples, they want a referee, not understanding. Want to be defined as "right"

Must determine the payoffs you are giving people for how they treat you. Is it healthy?

Even a long-standing pattern can be changed, but you can expect change to be resisted

Must be negotiated from a position of strength, requiring knowledge and resolve

If you cave in the behavior is reinforced

Acting as a victim or basing a plea on guilt will fail. Guilt is often used to resist change

LL 9: The power of forgiveness

Look at what anger and resentment can do to you. You give up your power to someone you hate

Hate, anger, and resentment are the most powerful emotions, and most destructive

Like fire in a forest, they consume you. Destroy all ability to love, feel peace, other positives

The physiological reaction makes the whole body negative. Misery is inevitable

The emotions are so strong they will change who you are. They completely change your perspective

Others may behave wrongly toward you, but it is up to you how you react to that

It isn't about them, it's about you. Release yourself, not them

Recognize you are locked in a bond with them, and they are taking your power

Assignment 13: Identify those whom you need to forgive and do so

LL 10 You have to name it to claim it

With your life manager (you) decide exactly what it is you want. Be bold, but realistic

This sounds easy, but few really know. Most know what they don't want

Be sure to separate the means from the end. E.g. a job may be a means or an end

Indecision creates inaction. Most you'll ever get is what you ask for

Tough enough to get the world to give you what you know you want

Need to be careful to go for what really is important and lasting

Create what you want in your mind: see it, feel it, experience yourself enjoying it

What is the price you will pay to get it? How many ways are there to get it?

Assignment 14:

Once you have named it, put together a plan to claim it, and don't give it up

A Guided Tour of Your Life

Create a life strategy to achieve your goals

Diagnose your current life in each of the charted areas. Look at the whole you, to know self

The Seven Step Strategy
1. Express your goal in specific events or behaviors
2. Express your goal in measurable terms
3. Set a timeline
4. Set a goal you can control
5. Plan a strategy that will get you to your goal
6. Define your goal by steps
7. Create accountability, with positive and negative reinforcement

CHOICES

Manage your choices

The end result of your life is the sum of all your choices
   If you manage your choices, you will manage your life
   Learning what and how to choose is *most* important
Choose: Faith, strength, honesty, belief in self, optimism, love,
   goals and directions, to accept others, to make own decisions, to accept
   responsibility for yourself, to work for what you believe, to learn from
mistakes, to choose *consciously* for yourself, etc.
We have free agency. Using it in a self-directed way is a *choice*
   Manage self only by conscious control of every choice
   Anyone who is able--and willing--to *think* can do it
     Must have courage to change, to take control
   "If do what always done, will get what always gotten"
   Do you think things thru, work, and see them thru to a
   complete conclusion?
Who we are is the result of *all* our choices
   It takes conscious decision and effort to overcome bad ones
   By continual wrong choices we can even give up agency
"Highest levels of heaven are those who *choose* to be there"

Develop the right mental programs

We talk to ourselves all the time, what we *say* determines what we *are*. Make
a *choice* of being positive
Negative self-talk is deadly--subconscious accepts as true
   Always talk in first person, present tense to build good
   mental programs
     Talk not about what *is*, but what you *choose*
     Create positive programs in your brain
     e.g. items in first paragraph: I *am* strong. I *am* optimistic
What we continually think about creates patterns in our brain
   Consciously consider: What do I talk to myself about?
   The strongest patterns you've created set your choices
   Patterns create mental programs, which determine how we act
     We are programmed by experience and others to make
     many wrong choices
     We can overcome old, and give ourselves new, programs
     Requires taking control of our thoughts for proper patterns
   Our subconscious will create any role we consciously give
Develop proper patterns by conscious thought and practice
   Always ask: 1] Is this a choice? 2] Decide: This choice is
   mine! 3] Obtain necessary info 4] Examine the

alternatives, then choose the best, even if it's not good

4] Say: My choice is ___. I made this choice because___ .

Build a habit. It becomes natural and stops procrastination

If we exercise the right to choose, we exercise the right to change. Choices begun today can reprogram our future

Our pattern of choices add up to 1 of 3 programs:

1] Build us up, 2] tear us down, 3] stay even

Examine own patterns and determine which of 3 you are

Look at each area of life

To become Pattern 1: 1] Ask: Where am I now? 2] Is it working? 3] Look at others for models, good and bad 4] Recognize own negative choices and patterns 5] Make a list of choices that would improve your patterns 6] Set goals for change 7] Begin changing *now* 8] Assess progress 9] Recognize and reward your successes

Choose!

For several reasons, we often fail to make choices we should:

Unclear goals, unclear self-image = unclear choices and failure. Remember:

All your little choices add up to you

Sometimes fail to recognize them as choices

Brain on autopilot: don't even realize choice is being made

Sometimes don't know what we should do, or how

Requires a conscious decision for self-education

Sometimes just not willing or afraid to make right choice

"Do what is right, let the consequence follow"

Society teaches us not to think--keep doing it the old way

Want us to be a school of fish: same speed and direction

3/4ths of our initial total programming is like this

If want to make better choices, must learn to *think*

Exercise agency, make *conscious* choices

Ask: What subconscious programs are making my choices?

Practicing on all the little choices sets up the big ones

Remember, when you have a problem, if you face it and make a decision you will feel better

Every primary choice requires supporting choices

All must be reviewed, determined, and carried out

If fail to do so, primary choice will fail

Write down primary and supporting choices for big decisions

They form a team

Primary choice sets the goal, supporting ones get the job done

One of our choices is our attitude

Ask: How do I feel? How would I like to feel? How do I *choose* to feel?

How we feel about anything is a choice of attitude
   Prove this by observing others: Attitudes vary even when
   circumstances don't. It is always the sum of their choices
Quichrbichn! We make our attitude worse by complaining
   May seem a harmless habit--(and there's lots to fuss about)
   But creates damaging mental programs imprinted on mind
   It reduces energy and affects attitude. It attracts negativity
   It accomplishes nothing, and makes you miss any good
    A bad event can ruin whole day--if choose to let it
   Have limited time and energy. Use to complain or achieve
   Choose to complain only if it will do some good
    Choosing not to complain is being an adult
Emotional choices are usually wrong
   Reason is overcome by feeling, e.g. anger, fear, passion
   1] Recognize the danger 2] practice objectivity 3] put off the
decision 4] control emotions (Great servants, but lousy
masters)
Actions (except involuntary ones) are always a choice
   Ask: What am I doing? What would I like to do? What do I
   choose to do?
   Want to know what choices you've made? How effective?
    Look at where you are in life
Many believe happiness, love, success, are fate, circumstances, or luck [The
kind of people who buy lottery tickets]
   Like everything else, these are *choices*: 3 of most important
   If don't believe so, then failing to accept responsibility
Happiness is an attitude. Attitudes are always up to you:
   Happiness is therefore always a choice
   Lincoln: "Most people as happy as make up mind to be"
   Each morning, *choose* to be happy today--and keep doing it
    Seems to be easy for some; impossible for others
May not be able to change circumstances, but can change
attitude
   Then, maybe, you can change your circumstances
   Can certainly do best with given set of circumstances
   Success, and happiness, defined and determined by that
Feeling of being in love always destroyed by realities of living
   The fireworks and the bells always die
   Must make the choice to *make* it work--self-responsibility
   Choose to respect and love, and to be respected and loved
   Make the necessary supporting choices
    How will you love? What will you give to get it?
    Are you willing to pay the price?

No one can achieve success automatically or easily
  Society programs us to be mediocre; tells us what *can't* do
    Must choose to remake the program. It is a *choice*
    If don't make conscious choice, then choose to fail
  Start believing--and telling self--what can do. Kill negatives
    Believe and choose: I *can!*
  Decide: Primary choice, supporting choices, price will pay

A Plan for Choosing

Look at the choices you make--imagine what new ones could do
in your life!
Ask yourself: "Who am I? What do I want?" What will it take?
  What price am I willing to pay?
  Are the things I want what are really important and fulfilling?
Write down primary and supporting choices in each of the following: My
family. My home. My personal relationships. My education (formal and
informal). My career. My income and money management. My other goals
and self-expectations. My health, fitness, and appearance. My spare time. My
happiness. My spirituality. My service to others. My attitude. My friendliness.
My self esteem. My personal style. My problem solving. My faith. My
thoughts. Other important areas.
Remember to work and balance all the following: spiritual, mental, emotional,
social, physical
Take control! Consciously define your choices
  Write new choices on 3 x 5 cards, carry, and read
  No one can do it but you. So do it!
As Kimball said: ***Do it! Do it right! Do it right now!***

How To Do What You Want To Do
-THE ART OF SELF DISCIPLINE   -Paul A Hauck

Preface: This is the last in a series of four books:
1. Depression: Usually results from self-blame, self-pity, other-pity
2. Hostility: Frustration and anger from a] I *must* have my own way
   b] People are bad and don't give me what I want
3. Fear: Apprehension and worry result from obsessing on concerns
4. Self Discipline: Without self discipline cannot overcome the others
   No maturity or success without it. Cannot get what you want
   Success requires doing often what you don't want to do

Three Obstacles To Self Discipline
Used to getting things too easily. Face it: It's a damn tough world
   Demand immediate satisfaction, and unwilling to defer gratification
   Expect the world should be different, and refuse to face reality
   Unwilling to work hard to plow thru the muck to get to the good stuff
Perfectionism: If it can't be perfect, won't do it
   More important to do, than to do well. Only disgrace is *not trying*
      Not: "If it can't be done well it shouldn't be done at all"
      Start and finish—that is how to define success, and to overcome
Feelings of inferiority: Should judge self by progress, not performance
   Stop caring about winning, and just play for the fun of the game
   Put pressure on the effort, not the outcome

Techniques of Self Discipline
Prioritize, and finish one job before starting next—have tunnel vision
Set specific goals—long term and short. *Do* them before a reward
   Never allow pleasure before work
   Make notes and to-do lists. Don't rely on memory
Just get started, especially if stoked, but even if not
Nibble at big jobs—break them into many small jobs
Just keep plugging! It may seem interminable, but it will get done
   The tortoise always beats the hare in the long run
   Be stoical—endure discomfort, boredom, pain, etc
      People who hide from pain receive the most pain
Associate with people who are disciplined and are models
Burn bridges to remove alternatives
Take risk: Failure is not a catastrophe: can't learn without
Don't watch, do. Do anything not excessively dangerous
Any time you slip, force yourself to make up for it *and* pay a price
Force yourself to cool down before doing something impetuous
   Good salespeople will fight this—for a reason

HOW TO WIN FRIENDS AND INFLUENCE PEOPLE
--Dale Carnegie

[Note: When I taught negotiation I said that you frequently can either get what makes you feel good or you can get what you want. Ego is the problem. To get what you want, ego *must* be subordinated, which requires humility and sound self esteem. Carnegie's famous book *HOW TO WIN FRIENDS AND INFLUENCE PEOPLE* offers specific techniques and has many examples. To be most effective, these principles must be followed as a matter of *character*, not as manipulative *techniques*. Following these principles requires acting differently from others and differently from natural inclinations. Perhaps the greatest leadership is to be able to practice these principles on oneself! While these skills are being developed, spend some time at the end of each day reviewing this outline and events of the day. Particularly analyze objectively your failures. How badly do you want to succeed at human relations?]

FUNDAMENTAL TECHNIQUES FOR DEALING WITH PEOPLE
Always **look for ways to give others honest and sincere appreciation**
The thing people want most is to feel important
>How you get a feeling of importance tells what your character is
>People even go insane to feel important

Sincere, accurate appreciation is the most effective way to make people feel important

Nourish their self-esteem--share their accomplishments and keep silent about your own
>Speak ill of no one, and all the good you know of everyone
>Flattery will not work--praise must be sincere and realistic

Practice by trying to have a positive effect on every person you meet
Never **criticize or condemn others**
All it does is cause resentment and kill desire

People will only make excuses when put on the defensive

Be humble: forgive and try to understand others. Remember:
>Everyone has a story
>If you will learn their story it's almost impossible not to like and respect them

Focus on what should be done, not on what is wrong
Arouse in others an eager want
Everything people do is because they want something

Only way to get anyone to do anything is if they want to
>Seek pleasure or avoiding pain. Former is much more motivating
>Show them how to get what *they* want, not what *you* want

Get to the other person's point of view to find what they want
>Try to get people to do something without ever talking

about what you want

Plant an idea and let them take the credit

TO MAKE OTHER PEOPLE LIKE YOU

Smile: It says, "I like you, I am glad to see you"

It can even be "seen" over the phone

Try to brighten others' lives

Make doing what you do fun

Force yourself to smile--feeling *follows* action

Find a way to be grateful for your circumstances, whatever they are

Become genuinely interested in others

People are not interested in you, only in themselves

People like those who are interested in them

Be *grateful* when people give you their time and attention

Be as friendly as a dog, and sympathetic and helpful

Remember a person's name is the sweetest sound

Make the effort to hear, learn, remember, and use it

Be a good listener; encourage them to talk about themselves and their interests

Be interested in what they are interested in

"Talk to people about themselves; they will listen for hours" -Disraeli

Listen intently, actively, and with concentration--let them do most of the talking

Do not interrupt, contradict, correct, wander, or focus on what you want to say next

Be a sounding board when needed: Better than giving advice

Make others feel important, sincerely

People's deepest need. In all interactions try to fill it. Show respect for everyone

Everyone is superior in some way. Find it and compliment it

Look for things to overtly admire by being sincerely interested in other people

Do not try to impress with your own accomplishments

TO WIN PEOPLE TO YOUR WAY OF THINKING

Begin in a quiet, soft-spoken, friendly way even when there is conflict

Smooth controversy by emphasizing points of agreement and keeping a sense of humor

Talk in terms of their interests, to develop rapport, before asking for anything

Lead, don't drive. Aggressiveness does not lead to agreement

Let others do a great deal of the talking

When they recognize you really want to know their ideas they will appreciate it and open up

Encourage them to come up with arguments pro and con and weigh them for

themselves
    Plant an idea and let them develop it and feel it is theirs
    Don't ram your ideas down others' throats. People don't like being "sold"
    Ask others for advice
Get people saying "Yes"
    Start with the things on which they agree. Get as many "yes" answers as possible
    Discuss their point of view and desires
Never **argue**
    You can't win an argument. Proving someone wrong won't make them like you
        Jesus said, "Agree with thine adversary quickly"
    Show respect for them and their opinions. Never say "You're wrong"
        When told wrong, people want to argue, not agree
            A look or intonation is as bad as words
        Find a way to demonstrate someone is wrong without
    actually saying so
            e.g. Socratean method: ask questions that lead to the answer
        Try honestly to see things from their point of view
            Even when wrong, others don't think they are. Find why think and act as do
        Let the other person save face. You have no right to damage another's self respect
    Agree you may be wrong and avoid all dogmatic or inflammatory statements
        Your open-mindedness can open the other's mind
        Minds can be changed only by gentle effort
        Understand others' opinions fully before making a judgment
    To keep disagreement from becoming argument:
• Welcome the disagreement--there'd be no progress if everyone always agreed!
• Sincerely thank them for their interest
• Distrust your own first impression--and say so
• Control your temper
• Emphasize areas of agreement; minimize disagreement
• Admit errors quickly, it shows courage and character
• Provide cooling down time for both to think; postpone the decision
• If they start yelling, let them get it out of their system, without over-reaction
• Keep listening to understand their point of view
• Express sympathy for their concerns, ideas, desires, and problems
Sincerely say: "I don't blame you for thinking and feeling as you do. If I were you I am sure that I would also"
    People crave sympathy; give it to them

TO BE A LEADER

When discipline is necessary, **begin with praise and honest appreciation**

Do not end a compliment with "but", always use "and" as a
conjunction

Call attention to mistakes indirectly

Talk about how to improve, not what is wrong

Show humility and fairness by talking about your own mistakes first

Instead of giving orders ask questions and give suggestions

Stimulate creativity and teamwork

Frame the request so it emphasizes the benefits to them

Praise the slightest improvement and every improvement

Use praise instead of criticism--reinforce positive behavior

Good things are reinforced and bad things will atrophy

To be credible, praise must be realistic, not flattery

Make the fault seem easy to correct

Praise things done right and minimize number and magnitude of errors

Do not tell anyone they have no aptitude for something--
it destroys incentive and self esteem

Give others a reputation to live up to. Have high expectations

They must respect you and know that you respect their ability

"Treat a person as he is, and he will remain as he is, but treat him as he can
and ought to be and he will become such"

Appeal to nobler motives

People usually have two reasons: One that sounds good and the real one

Help them think of the one that sounds good; Deemphasize the other

Throw down a challenge

All have fears, overcome them by challenge

Stimulate competition (with self and others), as a desire to excel

Dramatize

Stating something is not enough; use showmanship, get attention

"A picture is worth a thousand words"

BRINGING OUT THE BEST IN PEOPLE

--McGinnis

Goal is not to make lazy people industrious--it can't be done
   Rather to channel energies of energetic people
   There must be an inner drive already there
   Not manipulation, but persuasion to work in own best interest
   Find goals good for all and develop a "partnership"
Success depends more on leadership than hard work
   Success always requires leverage
     Leader must be a working psychologist
     Spend the time organizing and motivating--leverage
     Success must occur through the group for best effect
   Positive mental set of the group generates enthusiasm
      Enthusiasm feeds on itself until "critical mass" occurs, like a nuclear
reaction
     Strongly shared values and objectives provides a "culture"
     An extra 10% from each person is difference between failure and success

COMMIT TO EXCELLENCE AND EXPECT THE BEST

   Have strict core values--build team which supports
   Encourage pride in a good job; they buy in or get out
     Loose standards say its not worth caring about
     Stay with them and push--raise hell if not done
   Reprimand 1) immediately 2) confirm facts 3) be specific
   4) show feelings. *Allow* them to be unhappy with you
     Set the standard for each goal and make it clear
      People want to do a good job
   Attitude: the best is always yet to be done
   Create environment where people can do all they are capable
     Believe in the best
     A person is as good as the best he's ever done
   Build on people's strengths; deemphasize weaknesses
     Help them to succeed--concentrate on this
     Great ability is the ability to recognize ability
   Difficulty should be a challenge--struggle excites and inspires
     People long for a cause--try to create causes
      A cause will overcome boredom and lack of focus
     Do not intimidate or ask the impossible
     Provide for a series of successes
   Goals must be challenging but realistic
     Graded progression provides for feedback

MOTIVATION

Start from where the person *is,* not where they ought to be
Help people recognize what they want and how to get it
Use two-way communication
Must know the person and his values--everyone is different
Dig for needs and wants--these are in constant flux
Continuously seek to better understand people dealt with
People will explain how to motivate them if talk to enough
Help people set goals, plan, and then achieve the plan
Encourage big dreams and write down goals
Work to develop their ideas which you can support
Help people clarify their goals which are mutual
In effect, join *their* bandwagon
Goals must fit the group effort, and be very specific
Divergence from goal will energize correction
Same stimulus as hunger or frustration
Get commitment from individuals to support the group
Be certain public declaration only on positive concepts
Treat negatives by ignoring--addressing only reinforces
Maintenance of perceived self is basis of all behavior
Get them started
Attitudes follow behavior
Get a small commitment; later ask for larger, congruent
one--it supports the new self-image
Use models of success
Models may be from outside or inside the group
Stories of conflict, struggle, success
These stir feelings and change attitudes
Prove achievement is within reach
Create visual images of success
Have people relive own successes
Small Successes Lead to Bigger Ones
Repeater tendency: success breeds success
Look for successes--even small ones--and encourage
Develop the art of praise to reinforce desired behavior
Make gratitude a habit; employees, customers, etc.
People starve for appreciation
Create a winning environment
Develop systems to reinforce winning
Poor companies: less than half meet company's goals.
Good companies: most do.
Use: public commendations, give something tangible, every success is
a celebration, put it in writing if really exceptional, be specific (this also
reinforces). Do this for customers too.

Too much reward weakens motivation
Don't create reinforcement junkies
Praise the process as well as the result
E.g.:   Someone trying hard may not be succeeding

TEAMWORK
Key is to draw people to the group, more than to the leader
Most work best in a team
Mutual loyalty develops need to belong: reward cooperation
Assign high value to communication
Group takes responsibility for own standards
Group must believe leader puts their needs first
Must be genuinely caring--develop relationship of trust
If so, will even put up with an autocrat
Share discomfort, danger
Be consistent, keep your word, treat people fairly
Absolutely never betray a trust
Breach is fastest demoralizer
Individual must know he's part of group, but still an individual
The individual must count (e.g., if you salvage one employee, it is noted by all)
Have fun--take time to keep people laughing; go away together
Competition
Instinct to compete born in most people; strong tool for motivation, but use sparingly
Encourage excelling, not beating
Use comparisons to inspire, not criticize
Emotions provide great drive
Anger, fear, etc.--but use with care
Must be legitimate: injustice, wrong, etc.
Provide focus and energy and pull people together

MANAGE FAILURE
Ability to deal with failure varies extremely among people
Fear of failure kills drive
Failure inevitable--must be able to remotivate after
Ability to fail is critical to success
Be aware of failure and have a plan to counteract it
People must know failure is not fatal
Responsibility but not blame
E.g. shift jobs, assign task that allows success, etc.
Plan must fit circumstances and person
Praise and Reprimand
Use both, however negative must also include instruction
Do not be punitive or mean--but be bloody direct

Must fear consequences of actions--not you
Be tough but fair; show legitimate emotions
Do not procrastinate reproof--do it immediately
If privileges removed, do so for only short time
Provide means to earn back
Purpose not to control but to guide
Point out consequences and choices
Use guilt carefully and infrequently
Troublemakers
Have an allowance for storms
A lot easier to bank a fire than build one
The stronger the group, the more likely conflict will occur
Absorb others' complaints--let it ventilate up, not out
Know when to step in
Appeal to people's best side
Get to reasons: real one v. one stated
Ask for help, rather than dictating
Allow for some strange behavior
Ask self: "Is it really damaging"
Weigh contribution: sometimes life just too short to
deal with someone; sometimes they're worth the
problem

LEADERSHIP

Keys: 1) know the people 2) generate excitement
Enthusiasm is the flywheel which carries saw through
knots
A certain excessiveness is necessary. Be intense.
Don't be "one of the boys": a little eccentricity even helps
Think bold--but act. Be able to communicate the dream in a
big picture. Get people fired up. Take risks.
Take criticism well, no matter how it stings. Beware hubris.
Be certain everyone is getting full value
Keep own motivation high--that is a *choice*
Be really committed to the program
Monitor ideas coming into your mind--kill negative ones
Associate with successful, positive people
Plan goals in writing and continually review
Helping others can be life's greatest happiness
Be future oriented
Love it, dream it, talk it--the best is still ahead!

EXCERPTS RE: RAISING A STRONG-WILLED CHILD

"PARENTING" - from 10/01 "Psychology Today"- Azerad and Chance
The rise in outrageous behavior among children is unique to America
    Children in other industrial cultures are not rude, whiny, or violent
    Up to 25% of American children are diagnosed with ADHD
    Such children cannot be happy or feel good about themselves
    Such behavior predicts serious problems in later life
A major reason for children running amok is good-faith misplaced adult attention
    Parents are 5 times more likely to pay attention to bad behavior rather than good
    Children crave attention, even if negative, so the behavior parents pay attention to is reinforced
        Ironically, even discipline often reinforces bad behavior
Current child-rearing views result from philosophies of supposed "experts"
    Spock, Brazleton, Turecki, Greene
    Most child psychotherapy is an incompetent ripoff, according to R. Barden, PhD, JD
        Urge parents to hold, soothe, and explain to children who misbehave
        Encourage useless psychotherapy, with the child endlessly talking out the problem
        Child becomes convinced, from all the attention, that the problem is overwhelmingly serious
        Unintentionally encourages doing what gets noticed, so bad behavior is reinforced
Paying attention to good behavior, rather than bad, is difficult but necessary
    Unless really serious, the result of a real problem, or an issue of safety, ignore bad behavior
        Such as howling
    Be specifically on alert for good behavior, and reinforce it by compliments
        Point out they acted like an adult and, immediately after the praise, spend some time with them
        Remember to again reinforce the good behavior by praise some time after the event
        Never mix criticism in with praise
If safety is an issue or behavior is extreme, call a timeout
    Timeouts must be extremely boring, unrewarding, and consistent to be effective
- State simply the proscribed behavior. Do not discuss it
- Sit child in a chair facing the wall
- Be sure he stays in the chair at least 3 full minutes. The parent must be

in control
- Keep putting him back, and enforce with physical pain, if necessary
- Be sure he is behaving before releasing

THE STRONG-WILLED CHILD -by Dr James Dobson, 1978

Studies show the best parents excel in 3 key areas. They: 1] Effectively design and organize their children's environment, 2] Communicate well with their children, and permit interruptions by their children for up to 30 seconds, essentially any time, 3] Discipline firmly, while showing great love and affection. The child *must* get the message: "I love you more than anything, and because I love you I must teach you to obey me, for your happiness and safety, and that of others".

1. Just as animals test a human's authority, so must every child, particularly a strong-willed child

In schools, the most-loved teachers are the ones who love children, but are firm disciplinarians

Children respect strength and courage, and require their parents to prove they have it

Otherwise, children totally disrespect their parents, and will do everything to disobey

They are inexorable in the contest of wills, and continually work to wear their parents down

Everyone is miserable, including the child, and it is not something the child will "grow out of"

The child's will must not be broken, but he must be taught self control

Effective discipline requires love, lack of anger, firmness, consistency, and careful balance

The longer one waits to begin teaching discipline, the more difficult and frustrating it will be

Even Spock supported this view. He has been misquoted by all the modern liberal permissivists

He said permissiveness, even if well-motivated, makes an out-of-control child inevitable

Failure to learn to behave, ironically, absolutely destroys a child's self esteem

Wonders why his parents don't love him enough to protect him from himself

Grows up hating his parents and the world for never teaching him to control himself

Creates permanent misery in the home, and plants the seeds of permanent disaster for himself

The up side for the strong-willed child is, if he learns self control, he has great potential to achieve

2. *The most important distinction in child discipline is determining the child's*

motivation

Decide whether the misbehavior is childish error, or is intentional, willful, and defiant

Permissive psychology only recognizes and deals with the former; pretends latter doesn't exist

In the former case, i.e. childish error, discussion, illustration, and example are effective discipline

In the latter case, they *never* are – action is *required*: As long as you talk, the child will resist

Defiant children only become obedient when they know some serious action is about to occur

Talking is a waste of time, and is counterproductive: the child will engage in endless dialog

A child responds positively to anger and yelling only if he knows the next step is action

Children recognize anger as weakness, totally disrespect it, and learn just how far to push

For defiance, parents usually resort to action only as a *final* step, after frustration is unbearable

The important key is not to talk, but to act, and to act *immediately*

Parental frustration is avoided, discipline is more effective and can be less severe

Appropriate actions which may be taken include:

Require the child to sit in a chair facing the wall for a period of time, one minute per year old

It has to be long enough for him to get really bored and unhappy, and he must stay there

If he won't stay, then he has no respect for you – and more drastic action is needed

Take away something he wants – and keep taking things till he behaves or has nothing to do

Send him to bed early, with nothing to do – and make him stay there

If nothing less works, then pain is required

Pinch hard on top of the shoulder muscle – it really hurts, but no damage

Spank. Remember, this is only used – and necessary – for deliberate, willful, disobedience

After discipline, hug him and tell him you love him – but repeat discipline as often as required

3. Guidelines for parents to shape the will, without damaging the spirit

• Write out in detail the exact problem, the rules, and the disciplinary plan

• Recognize and accept responsibility that the parent *must* be the one ultimately in control

- Establish the rules firmly, but with as broad latitude as possible, to allow self-responsibility
- Allow children, within reason, to suffer the natural consequences of mistakes and misbehavior
- There are so many "No"s for children, try to have as many "Yes"s as possible
- Define reasonable boundaries before enforcing them. Avoid impossible demands
- When the child misbehaves, always distinguish whether the act is irresponsible or is willful
- When faced with willful behavior *act immediately*, decisively, and confidently
- Reassure, love, and teach after the discipline, as soon as the child will accept it
- Perfect discipline is not required. Parents need to act as a unit, and do it right most of the time
- The bottom line: Parents must succeed, or they will raise out-of-control children who will destroy themselves, and life will be miserable for everyone during the process.

MEND THE BROKEN BOND, by Dr Phil, 9/26/07, with Dr Frank Lawlis

Childhood should be joyous, and almost all parents love their children and have good intentions

Frequently, however, the methods parents use in discipline are wrong, tho well-intended

The most serious situations are shown by a child's self-injury, e.g. banging head on wall

> Results when child feels deeply insecure, lack of control, lack of communication

> Self-injury is used as a distraction from mental pain—the physical pain seems less

Have to try to look at the child's world thru the child's eyes, and deal appropriately

> Parents are large and intimidating and, for good or bad, are the standard for behavior

>> Children try to emulate their parents, so they act as they see them act

>>> Loud, demanding, arbitrary, aggressive action is usually a mirror of the parents

>>> Parents must remain calm, rational, negotiable; it's not a battle of the wills

Children need to feel they have control in their world, or they become insecure

> In their own way, they will fight for a sense of control if it is not provided

to them

Need to feel they have their fair share of parents' time and attention

Develop a practice of reinforcing good behavior, disciplining only when absolutely must   Do not demand absolute control, but teach children they have the right to negotiate with you

Teach them, by experience, they get more by cooperation and negotiation than tantrums

Battles of the will teach them just the opposite

Children need to feel there is real communication, and their feelings are fairly considered

Children *must* know that parents understand just how intensely bad they may be feeling

They do not have adequate words to express their feelings, so they act them out in tantrums

Teach them the words for negative feelings and encourage them to express themselves

[There is a chart for this which shows negative faces and gives a word for each]

Make sure you have mutual eye contact when talking, especially during tantrums

Make sure they know you are listening, understand, and are giving fair consideration

Even if you don't always, of course, give them what they want

Use hand gestures, etc to help express what children have difficulty understanding

EXAMPLES
Dr Phil Interview 8/31/04

Interviewed a couple who had a daughter, age 7, who refused to behave. Hurt her siblings, pitched fits, took anything she wanted. Parents had tried everything, including spanking, and had finally caved in to her stronger will. Phil's first point: You cannot solve a problem unless you are willing to admit it exists. Unless there is a serious medical condition, parents are always the problem with child behavior. In this case, the Mother has the role of enforcer. When Dad comes home, he is tired(!), and just wants to play with the kids. Daughter knows all she has to do is survive till Dad gets home, and all the discipline will go out the window. He disciplines sometimes, but is absolutely inconsistent, and the daughter treats her Mother, who is doing all she can, with contempt because the Father allows it. The daughter must have an absolute signal there are rules and they are inviolable, except with immediate, serious penalties, which will be enforced every time by both parents as a unit. Father wants to enjoy his kids, but this is not about the Father's wants, it is about the daughter's needs, and there will be terrible consequences for the daughter in the future if those needs for discipline aren't met.

Dr John Rosemond, PBS Program, 8/29/04 [Author of *Parenting the Strong-Willed Child*]

Dr Rosemond was told of a child who had terrorized his family from infancy, until he was able to broaden his horizons by terrorizing the school. The parents finally came to Dr Rosemond when he was in fifth grade because he was going to be permanently expelled unless put on "meds" for "ADHD". He had them lock the kid *out* of his room for a month. *All* his possessions were inside, and he was allowed in only once a day to get clothes. He wanted to know where to sleep, and was given a blanket and told to find a couch. He was also told that every time there was a complaint about him, from school or other sources, he would have a day added on the calendar. The middle of the second week, there was a call from the child's teacher. Wanted to thank them for finally admitting the kid had ADHD and putting him on medication. . . . .

Others

A woman from church had kids who were out of control. She obstinately insisted the most important principle was that they knew unquestionably that she loved them, and that discipline was counterproductive to that. Every one grew up to be a disaster, with two of them in prison.

One of my sons, after he was an adult, said, "Dad, when I was in high school you gave us kids a beater car to drive. Some of my friends' parents gave them hot new cars, and my classmates used to tease me about having to drive a beater when my Dad had a stable of really great sports cars. It was a little embarrassing at the time, but I handled it O.K. My friends who were given everything grew up to expect everything should still be given them, and they are pretty worthless. You taught me that if I wanted something I would have to earn it, and I owe my success to that lesson. Thank you!"

A friend had a nearly uncontrollable stepson, and home life was an uproar. His mother could not, or would not, control him and his father refused to take any responsibility, letting him run wild whenever the boy was at his house. The stepfather said to me, "I can't take any more. I'm going to send him to live with his father". I told him, "You are the only source of discipline that kid has ever had. I know it's tough, and the constant battle has completely worn you out, but did you ever stop to think you're not just the best chance that kid has, you're the *only* chance?" He decided not to give up, and did the best he could, and the boy finally learned to control himself and to direct all that energy toward positive objectives. He is now a well-mannered, successful adult.

WHY MARRIAGES SUCCEED

John Gottman

Book is based on empirical data from studies of 2000 marriages
   Found much conventional wisdom is wrong
   Similarities do not safeguard against divorce
   Conflict does not necessarily lead to divorce
   Anger is not a negative! It is necessary to a healthy marriage
     It is how it is handled, not its existence. Value the struggles!
     Lasting marriage results from resolution of inevitable conflicts
     People who do not fight are likely in an unhappy marriage
     Final solution is less important than communicating
   Most important: The 5:1 ratio; Common arguing style
Women are the emotional leaders in marriage
   Life conditions them to express, men to repress
   Women can't expect same verbal intimacy from husband as friend
     Have unrealistic expectations of marriage
     It is no one's "job" to make the other happy
   It's usually the wife who begins the negative process
     Attack causes withdrawal, attacks increase, w'drawal increases
   Women tend to be too emotional, men too rational
     In happy marriages this distinction is reduced
       Men must learn not to avoid conflict, but to embrace anger
         Recognize attack is not personal; Accept even if don't agree
       Women must confront gently, criticize less, stop mind reading
       Both must learn more acceptance and treat respectfully
Successful marriages invariably use "repair mechanisms" in conflicts
   Consciously and intentionally given and accepted to soothe
     Express attention and affection, even if forced
     Not necessarily done in a conciliatory tone, but they are done
     May even be rude, but show involved, not withdrawing
   Maintain eye contact, show you're listening
   Try to keep a sense of humor
   At times don't say anything, just listen
   Do not issue ultimatums or force issues
   Talk about *how* you are talking and arguing
   Consciously agree to look for resolutions
The Magic Ratio: 5 to 1
   5 positive strokes given by each for every negative hit
   Most important determinant to successful marriage
   Negatives are *necessary* to a healthy marriage
     Better than 5 to 1 is not good!

There always will be differences, and these must be dealt with
Couples without conflict likely to end in divorce
One thing negatives do is reduce boredom and keep up passion!
Positives: Show interest, affection, caring, appreciation,
concern, empathy, acceptance, joke, share joy
In healthy marriages a "balance thermostat" kicks in for conflict
Positives—repair mechanisms—given, even if forced
They are carried and received by basic love and respect
Shown by gestures, eye contact, face, as well as words
Evidenced by positive comments to third parties about spouse
Marriages seem to settle into 1 of 5 styles—3 healthy, 2 not
Closer the marriage fits 1 of the 3, more likely to succeed
2 keys determine success: 5 to 1 ratio, agree on common style
Validating Style: Listen, understand, accept even if don't agree
Little hostility, much respect and persuasion, moderate emotion
Each other's best friend and good companion
Do a lot of active listening, mutual supporting
Much good faith and compromise to resolve conflicts
The classic ideal of a good marriage
Volatile Style: Very open about expressing negative feelings
Open and honest, often to the point of causing pain
Tease a lot, sometimes causing hurt; compete continually
Bicker over every minor thing, each trying to persuade
Interrupt rather than try to understand
See selves as both nurturing and expressive
But these serve to fuel the positives in the relationship
Many more negatives, but also many more positives
A lot of passion in the marriage—love "making up"
See selves as independent equals, interrupt each other often
Each needs a lot of personal space and independence
Avoidant Style: Minimize conflict, make light of differences
Little attempt made to solve issues: "agree to disagree"
Do not talk things out: Sweep conflicts under carpet and ignore
Focus on shared vision of a strong marriage
Bond so strong can overlook disagreement
Have least emotion and passion of 3 types
More the partners' natural styles are same, more likely to succeed
Serious conflicts occur if styles differ; permeates all arguments
Each has different way to argue, show love, handle emotions
Every conflict has problem of how to argue and relate
E.g. avoidant style is seen as dishonesty by a volatile
Must analyze differences and compromise a common style
Survival of the marriage depends on this

Volatile and avoidant most difficult
Key: Whatever else, criticism, contempt, defensiveness, stonewalling
absolutely *must* be avoided by *both*. I.e. address the symptoms
2 types unhealthy marriages:
   Hostile/engaged: Argue continually with great heat
      Name calling and sarcasm, but look at each other and listen
   Hostile/disengaged: Arguments hot, but do not look or listen
      Generally detached and emotionally uninvolved with each other
   Both types *invariably* characterized by a *specific* downward spiral
      Criticism, then Contempt and Defensiveness, then Stonewalling
      The 5 to 1 ratio is not maintained
      The cycle is more and more difficult to break as it continues
         Like a broken record, negative thoughts endlessly repetitive
         If near a solution to an argument, one will sabotage
   Healthy marriages can degenerate into one of these styles
      Danger signs: Can't remember why attracted, criticize to 3d
      parties in front of spouse, remember nothing good from past
   Criticism is general vs. complaints which are specific
      "You are a jerk" vs. "I don't like you yelling"
      Complaining is good, and needs to be addressed
         But complaints become criticism if they go unheeded
         Frustration will lead into the spiral
   Contempt is the intention to psychologically abuse partner
      Attack sense of self by verbal and non-verbal abuse
         Cannot even remember, do not communicate, any positives
      Use by insults, name calling, sarcasm, mockery, body language
         Done in front of 3d parties is absolute indicator of divorce
   Defensiveness is completely natural reaction to contempt, criticism
      Unfortunately, does not matter that you are right
      It obstructs communication and nothing is resolved
Evidenced by: denying responsibility, excuses, cross-complaints,
yes-butting, repetitions—getting mutually louder and more vitriolic
   Stonewalling is *habitually* refusing to listen to confrontation
      Stonewallers are just trying to be neutral and avoid conflict
      But partner becomes totally frustrated and wants to scream
      Absolutely destructive. 85% are men, pressed by women
This downward spiral eventually becomes cast in stone
   Feel like innocent victim: take no responsibility, take no action
   Focus on righteous indignation: have total contempt, want revenge
   Total emotional overload is a continual state
      Identified by high heart rate, shallow breathing, tenseness
   Become conditioned to respond irrationally
   Everything a confirmation of negative feelings—self-fulfilling prophecy

Blind to any evidence of good, totally mistrustful
Every conflict reinforces futility; no longer try to resolve things
Continuously rehearse negative thoughts, forget all positives
Final stage: Parallel lives in same house; complete isolation from spouse
If the spiral is not broken and reversed the relationship is over
Once spiral down is cast in stone, only way to break is tell spouse:
"I love you and am lonely without you" [Not bad other times!]
Must consciously, intensely, and mutually work on specific plan:
Calm down. Disengage and take time-outs when necessary
Agree in advance to stick to one complaint per argument
Agree to argue only 15 minutes at a time—but agree to argue
Argue formally: agenda, state positions, divide argument time,
establish alternatives, look for compromises, make a decision
Validate each other verbally and by body language
Volatiles must learn this. Must tone down, edit what they say
Must follow common rules of politeness. Force it if needed
Express good as well as bad; apologize and take responsibility if wrong
Look for, specifically express positives and areas of agreement
Do not be hyperrational or give advice; acknowledge feelings
Agree absolutely not to criticize or express contempt
Force yourself to complain about specific incident *only*
Do not use arguments as a way to retaliate
Listen and speak non-defensively. *Refuse* to defend yourself
Must force self not to, it only results in escalation
Look for the imbedded complaint and respond only to that
Overlearn these techniques so can use when stressed—practice!
Share happy times: children, recreation, hobbies, business, church, etc.

THE BATTLE OF THE SEXES

R C

["*" in the text indicates the most critical concepts for a successful relationship. These are summarized at the end.]

People talk a lot about the "Battle of the Sexes". It is probably *the* most universally popular topic; it is certainly among the most important. The relationship between men and women is not so much a *battle* as it is a *struggle*; a struggle to understand and be understood, a struggle to work out conflicts and get along; a struggle to please each other and be happy together. For one side to "win" the battle would be a loss for all—we need *all* to win! The benefits are enormous. The philosophy of Tao says everything is simple and natural, so go with the flow. But that is not the case with relationships in our complex society. Some of the concepts here defy reason, many are counterintuitive – and many violate inclination!

Dr Phil says there are 2 reasons marriages fail: Choosing the wrong partner, or sabotage by one or both. I think there is a third, larger and more important. Our two most important "jobs" are being a spouse and being a parent, and they are the two things for which we receive the least training. Society provides no real instruction or help—other than the (often poor) example of parents. The failure of my first marriage, to a person with whom I could have had the kind of relationship this composition describes, was entirely my fault. Though failure of my second marriage was not my fault (although I now recognize that is not entirely true), I finally realized that this is a complex as well as a serious matter, and that I needed to look into it seriously. So I did my usual routine when something has my attention: I studied and outlined two dozen books, I pondered, I made notes, and I talked at length with a noted Clinical Psychologist, Glade Birch. For example, when Glade told me about primal instincts, I realized how much I had misunderstood and, though in good faith, how many mistakes I had made. I said, "I've got to go think about this". I spent most of the next two days in thought.

The primary purpose of learning is not knowing but *doing*. Information is a tool, and it is a good tool to the extent it promotes effective action. I wrote this outline to organize my thoughts and notes on the subject, to create a good tool. It is written for my children, and I hope it will keep them from many of my mistakes. It draws heavily from things I read and was told. "SPISE", "CAST", "CARE", and "CLASS" are acronyms I developed to help remember. The "Faith" section was taken from thoughts in my book. Faith is critical: *Everything* is faith.

Relationships can be difficult, and are attacked from many sources. This is particularly true in our permissive, promiscuous society. The one thing worse than no relationship is a bad relationship. A mate must be selected carefully - one who is absolutely committed to marriage, who is honest, loyal, and mature, who will continue to grow with you, and who will remain always faithful through a long life together - and the relationship must be carefully and constantly nurtured. That ought to be fun! The purpose of this outline is to help make the selection and, over the years, develop the relationship. A relationship should bring the greatest satisfaction, happiness, and growth together. It all comes down to one simple principle: Each must want to be with the other more than just about anything else in the world.

Remember: this is an outline; you will need to ponder each point. I have written detailed outlines far shorter than this of whole books. The outline covers the entire process: dating, choosing a mate, getting along in marriage, and dealing with conflicts. Remember, too, that this is written from my own—limited—point of view. I am not a professional in this subject, and lack both breadth and depth of experience. But I've long said, "God save us from the professionals: they do it for money!" Amateurs do it for love: they are driven to understand. I hope this outline serves you well in your struggle and will save you from many of my blunders.

Dad

RELATIONSHIPS

Most things in life, once achieved, seem to lose value
    Only one thing in life can continue to grow in satisfaction
        That is associations with people
To love and be loved is a basic, deep human need
    People are social beings: need mate, family, friends
    Won't die without it, but cannot be entirely happy
*Relationship with one's spouse, including physical, emotional, spiritual, has potential to be the most satisfying relationship
    Instinctual—almost compulsory
    Like everything of value, it takes planning and work
        —but the rewards!
Falling in love [vs. being in love]:
Falling in love: An illusion will last forever, but max 2 years
    Admittedly wonderful if it happens in the beginning
        But not necessary for a happy, successful relationship
        More likely to be counter-productive: the wrong reason
    Physical (looks) and emotional "chemistry"
It is a feeling. It is self-centered. Some move from one relationship to the next, trying to keep the feeling
        Like buying a puppy, taking it to the pound when grown
            Then buying another puppy

The "grass is greener" syndrome
>It's greenest where it's nurtured—and it takes two

Also a *projection* of characteristics, needs, expectations
>E.g. a woman's "knight in shining armor"
>The reality never equals the daydream

"I love you" is often a weapon of relationships
>Men use to seduce, women to get commitment
>>Both use to get reassurance for own insecurities

>People of character, therefore, are often shy of saying it
>>Their partner can't understand, and resents this

>May also not say because not said to them when young
>>Must keep saying till comfortable

Being in love: Has the potential to last, and grow, forever
>Requires the elements of romantic love discussed later

Individually and as partners we must grow from dependence thru independence to interdependence
>Both must have the capacity for independence

>*More* than a feeling, it is a decision: one *wills* it
>>Have to be willing to, and pay, the price
>>Requires a *mutual* exercise of faith
>>A permanent, irrevocable *mutual* commitment

>No quitting when things get tough
>No quitting when the "feeling" is gone
>No quitting if you meet someone "better"
>Not dependency: "I need you"
>Not codependency: "I need you to need me"
>>One an enabler, the other dependant
>Not selfishness: "You need to make me happy"
>Not self-sacrifice: "I need to be a martyr"

1 Cor. 13:4-7 characterizes love:

Love endures long and is kind; envies not; boasts not, is not haughty, does not behave inappropriately, seeks not for advantage, is not easily provoked, thinks no evil; rejoices not in injustice but in truth; bears all things . . .

It is "The will to extend oneself to nurture one's own or another's spiritual growth" [*The Road Less Traveled*]
>A standard to evaluate own, and others', love

Requires time, attention, risk, service, responsibility, discipline

Leads to most satisfying growth and unity
>It wants what's best for the other [*Personality Types*]
>>It is what you do for someone else if you love them
>>For them to be strong and independent
>>Even if it risks the relationship

>It outlives lack of response, selfishness, mistakes

Never used to take what is not freely given
A choice to follow the second commandment
    For a specific and special "neighbor"
Each can be, for the other, the most wonderful person on earth
    During the honeymoon phase, it *seems* this way
    Over the years, this can become the reality
    She should be his biggest fan; he should be hers
    Admire the things each wants to be admired for
Women *need* romance, and the man must provide it
    If man can't, or won't, relationship *at best* mediocre
        Loses all potential intimate benefits
        "Romantic" is not something you *are*, but you *do*
    Must be done on her terms—make magic
        Doesn't require a lot, but must be continual
        Show [not tell] thinking of them. Create "you-and-me"
        Find ways to appeal to all 5 of the senses
        Use happy surprises; get her out of daily environment
        Pay attention to smallest details. Show thinking of them
            Show made an effort, e.g. clean the car before a date
        Appreciate her and have fun!
Love needs to be expressed in your partner's terms
    People express, and look for, love in different ways
    If it seems need can't be satisfied despite all your efforts
        May just be trying to give it in the wrong way
Five Love Languages, discussed by Chapman, include:
        Verbal, Quality time, Gifts, Service, Touch
        [I suspect there are others – including some sick ones]
    Love is discovering what spouse wants, and giving it
        This is *critical*, or may seem like a bottomless pit
            I.e. If whatever you do doesn't work, isn't enough
            If all efforts seem completely futile, unreciprocated
    Make a choice to do it, whether you feel like it or not
        If it doesn't come natural it is more loving if you do it
        Feelings *follow* choices and acts, as well as vice versa
    Look for the ways your spouse expresses love
        How they try to give shows how they want to receive
    Also, they may be giving love even tho you don't see it!
"Unconditional love" [in my opinion] does not exist
        Except, perhaps, by a mother for her baby
        Despite infinite love, God sends sinners to hell
        Even Jesus had his favorite disciple, the "one he loved"
Loving another on their own terms is closest
    It seems to them like unconditional love. Call it that

Too often, people date and marry beneath themselves [Tho, generally, good men seem to marry women better than they. On average, women seem to be better than men]

Marrying beneath oneself violates concepts of equity. Reasons:
Low self esteem, inadequate sense of own value
To have good self esteem must 1] have a clear Conscience, 2] be successful at Achieving worthwhile things, 3] give Service, 4] control any negative mental "Tapes"

Underdeveloped conscience is the sign of character defects

An overdeveloped conscience indicates neurosis

Most people try to build ego, based heavily on 2] and some 3]
No sense of who they are, own worth, where want to go

Can't soar with eagles if scratching with turkeys

Have not defined and committed to a value system

Consider: Where want to be in 5, 10, 20 years?
Good people, who are potential mates, seem unexciting

This is lack of maturity

Unrealistic, romantic desires interfere with a good choice

Nice guys, for example, don't seem "confident" enough

End up marrying someone "exciting" – who is a jerk
Have made no effort to prepare and to continue growing

Kind of person they might attract is not attracted

Need to be the best can be
"Bargain Hunters", looking for the best "deal"

Then want to switch when something "better" comes along
Looking in the wrong places (like bars)
Fooled by a phony (Anyone can fake it for a while)

"Bait and switch"
Just have to have someone in their lives at all times

Give up too soon in finding a good person

Women, particularly, often can't stand not to have a partner
Become pregnant
Prostitution: Marry for money, status, etc.
Michael Allred, BYU, lists love counterfeits

Baby love: Must be held. When one leaves, another is substituted

Toddler love: Highly possessive: "Mine!"

Elementary school love: Playing grownup, like dressing grownup

Middle school love: The label is what matters—need trophy and conquest
Both partners must be mentally healthy and mature, i.e. adults
Both must have stability and commitment

To deal with a lifetime of ups and downs
Are you willing to self-examine and work on your issues?

Will you admit them, and work to be your own best self?

You have to be healthy *together*
Everyone has some neuroses and insecurities
    Find out which and how bad
    Some have an emotional hole so deep you can never fill it
        Loving in the way they seek can go a long way
Men tend to be attracted to neurotic women
    Like the old song "Spooky"
    They seem interesting and exciting, never dull or boring
    Men's competitive nature as a hunter keeps them coming back
Neurotics, consciously or unconsciously, have a hundred ways to keep a guying playing the game "She loves me, she loves me not!" It goes back to the "Boy-girl theory"

PRIMAL INSTINCTS

People are not intelligent, rational, sophisticated beings
A relationship is not two independent people who choose to be together for mutual satisfaction (as I once thought)
    Basic instincts are powerful, unconscious, and primal
        They drive men and women to be together
        They are not based on reason
        Love is a basic, and powerful, human need
        Our feeling of self worth depends on relationship success
Man's instinct: Be a Provider and a Protector
    Needs to feel needed and trusted; needs to deserve this
    Providing for a woman gives confidence and fulfillment
    Needs to be accepted as is; big fear is incompetence as P&P
Hates being treated like a little boy: supervised, scolded, corrected, questioned, etc.
    Hates having a woman try to change him
        If she keeps telling him what to do, he's outta here!
        These motivated by her insecurities—must control them
    Man's role as a hunter carries into relationships
        His responsibility and propensity to take the initiative
        Woman's role is whether to respond, where to draw lines
            No gentleman will take "no" for "maybe"
Woman's instinct: Be worthy of love, to attract and keep P&P
    Needs to feel cherished, validated, fulfilled, protected
    Women are natural sacrificers
    Most happy when primal needs, i.e. security, are met
        Hates failure to have feelings validated
            Determinative of whether she trusts
        Hates lack of continual attention
            Needs time spent with her
            Continual expressions of love, in her language

Attacks at the level of primal instincts absolutely destructive
  E.g. a man who can't keep a job
    A woman who can't feel secure in keeping a mate
  Relationships depend on having these needs met
  Men and women don't understand their differences
    Try to give what they themselves want
    Don't need to give more, just what is needed
Some women stay with a guy who hits because he will also hit anyone who makes a move on her: "He loves me!"

WORKING THE SOCIAL ENVIRONMENT

Application to social gatherings, public places, telephone
  Make most of every situation, even if just for practice
  Problem often is not shyness, just knowing how and practice
Basic principles
  Attitude: Decide to do it and have fun; take risk. Can't eat you!
  Prepare in advance: Social skills, Goal, Plan, Approach,
    Conversation topics
  Chutzpah: Be confident and willing to hang it out there!
Charisma: Confidence, smile, eye contact [7 sec. on, 7 off], sincerity, listen actively
In social situations act like a "host", not a "ghost"
  Enter a room confidently, check it, walk up to someone
    Start with a wallflower, to make it easy. Give everyone a lift
  Meet everyone, make them comfortable, get others together
Relax and act confident, so others can relax – enjoy it!
  Like an athlete, try to get "in the zone", with energy
  Avoid big mistakes: E.g. aggressive, weird, bad jokes, bad dress
Learn your role as a guy or woman – how to dress, act, etc
Women hate "weirdness", bad breath, B.O., nose and ear hair
Is she interested?
  Make eye contact and hold too long. She will look away
    Subtly [no staring] see if she looks back in under a minute
  Smile [Don't grin or leer!], a little later nod, then *move*
    If you aren't confident, fake it. "Fake it till you make it"!
  Try to create love at first sight: Your looks, confidence, manner
    Women judge men by whether they can imagine kissing them
Introducing yourself
Say "Hi", state name and something relevant and neutral
  About you, them, the event, etc.
Women hate lines. Keep it light, simple, and sincere
Practice by just saying "Hi" to everyone you encounter
  The best pick-up line ever devised? Research proven!
  Lighten up and say, "Hi, I'm ___. May I join you?"

Simple, to the point, not banal, they must say "yes" or "no"
>If blown off, at least you indirectly paid a compliment!

Small talk
>Have 3 subjects selected and developed in advance
>>Saying almost *anything* is better than nothing
>>>But be creative not banal

Women complain men ask 5 things: Age, how long divorced, what work, # kids, # home. But they ask the same!
>>Listen to responses for keys: stepping stones to other subjects
>>>Remember details about them for conversation at later dates
>>>Ask "What's new since I saw you last?"

Be confident, sincere interest and total focus on them, empathy, light enthusiasm and humor, use their name often
>Use subtle body language to show they're irresistible
>Be positive, respectful, patient, appreciative, non-conflicting

Act "normal" – create trust. Never argue
>Notice something about them to compliment
>>Notice details about them, and ask for the story
>>Ask a polite open-end question and then develop it
>>>"Where've you thought about going in this lousy weather?"
>>Look for common areas: interests, background, etc.

Make creative misinterpretations and innuendos
>I.e. effective *light* flirting

Carry your end, and help them carry theirs
>People hard for you to talk to are also hard for others
>>Actually an advantage! With some planning and effort it's easy

Never interrupt or argue. Show genuine interest and develop trust

Watch the signs, particularly body language
>If you don't strike oil, stop boring

Breaking in on two or more [the larger the group, the safer]
>Avoid if 2 people are directly facing, close, and intense
>Watch for verbal cues and body language; try to work in slow
>If slightly know, can greet and act as if leaving, to see if invited

Moving on
>If "no deal", cut it quick and clean and go on to the next person
>E.g. "Nice talking to you", "Catch you later", "Guess we should mingle"
>If someone acts indifferent, insistent, or rude, just walk away
>>If someone rude won't take "No" for an answer, rudeness justified
>>>Some aggressive people take advantage of others' politeness

Moving ahead
>Be excellent in their presence—earn it
>Read all body language and verbal cues to see if it's reciprocated
>Ramp up eye contact, looking directly into their retina

Know her eye color!

Get into more serious subjects, to develop intimacy

    Ask about dreams, fears, ambitions, and emotions

    Get thru the social mask

Move from clichés and superficialities to personal questions, feelings, and "we"

    Judicious self-revelation can lead into mutual revelation

        It is amazing what people will tell you

        Build rapport, tell personal info about self—ask!

    Flirting is a requirement for developing intimacy

        Use words, humor, facial expressions, body language

        Early on especially, limit it to good-natured and friendly

        Be careful and ready to back off, even apologize

    Build momentum, but don't push it

        Emails, phone calls, dates, increased intimacy

        If anything intimate happens, call the woman the next day

        Otherwise she will feel used

The five-step process to intimacy

    The hotter the person, the better you have to play it!

Non-verbal signals [Eye contact, increasing over time], Verbal greeting, Turning toward each other [initially the heads], Touching [she first], Synchronization of movements

    Each must occur, and in this order

    Either can back off—or blow it—at any stage

Look for sign of readiness to close, and ask for a date, get a number

Getting someone to fall for you—in a nutshell:

2 Keys: 1] Find a way to get them really curious about you

      2] Learn and express how they are unique and special

"SOFTEN": Smile, Open posture, Face them, Touch, intense Eye contact, Nod and agree

If a guy, be a Southern Gentleman—they are all but extinct

Open doors, hold coat, walk on outside, stand when she does, swat the spiders, fight the battles, take the bullet

    All part of being a man. If don't want to do it, then be a fairy

THE DATING GAME

Have to get in the game if you hope to win

    They say all good things comes to those who wait

        The only thing waiting will get you is gray hair

        Go where they are, and keep going till you're comfortable

A game in the sense it has objectives, consequences—and rules

    A fact, whether one likes it or not

        Those who say they don't play games often are the worst!

        Don't be paranoid, but look out for those not in good faith

If you're not in good faith and honest, may "win" a really unsuitable, unhappy relationship

In a relationship the games should stop

The game is not necessarily bad, if played in good faith

If you refuse to play, or play badly, you will lose

Like basketball, got to know the rules and follow them

If don't, look foolish and cannot play effectively

Put your best foot forward

Dress, groom, and behave well

If a guy, always have a plan – creative, confident, and caring

"Whatcha wanna do?" won't cut it. Alternatives are good

Learn your role, as a guy or woman

You can't expect to be treated or respected as a lady or as a gentleman if you don't look and act like one

Trying to meet someone always carries the risk of rejection

Also the risk of having to rebuff another

Two possible attitudes:

1] "Sales" approach: Of every ___ you try, one will respond

Rejection is just a necessary part of the process

2] Take the risk only for people you believe you can really care about; it's not worth it for the others

Why give someone you aren't really interested in the satisfaction of rejecting you?

Why try to date someone you have no serious interest in?

All things of value entail risk – but evaluate and risk with care

Don't be paranoid or risk-averse, but do guard yourself

If there is a chance of physical risk, be particularly careful

If your heart gets broken, suffer a little – and then get over it

It's not going to kill you

Use displacement: Focus on something or someone else

The woman generally sets the pace in the relationship

Whether interested, how intimate to be and how quickly, when to kiss and how passionately, etc.

It's the man's job to initiate, but he has to read the signals

It's the woman's job to send the signals, and be consistent

Mostly this is done by body language

Whether to become acquainted, continue, intensify

Failure by her to do so may be ignorance or calculated

If she'd like to pursue it, but does not send the signals, she can't complain if it doesn't happen [And women today are allowed far more latitude than ever before]

If she doesn't want to, but sends the signals, she can't complain if it does happen!

There's a name for women who send mixed signals!
Creating romantic love requires "CARE"
1] Chemistry, 2] Amicability, 3] Respect, 4] Equity
If want someone, have to develop these in them
Each must be consciously worked on and maximized
People make decisions subjectively
They use reason to justify the decision. So cover both angles
Perception is often more important than reality
Chemistry
This is listed first as it is the element that usually starts it all
Particularly for a guy
A certain level of attractiveness is necessary. Beyond that there are things far
more important
Physical, but also emotional, attraction
Looks, grooming, personality, style, presence
If it's not there, *usually* nothing will substitute
Really attractive people usually agree it should be a 50-50 deal
They got the looks, so their partner should provide all the rest
Love at first sight?
Some psychologists argue the subconscious can identify traits in others,
beyond the physical, both negative and positive, that relate to attraction
between people (called "Imago match")
People tend to want what can't have—the "boy-girl theory"
People pursue what retreats
Anything too easy seems of little value
Be a challenge—but give hope, be a friend
Game: "If you want me enough, you'll keep trying"
But keep trying without *being* trying
Quit and walk away before becoming obnoxious
Use body language to show you're attracted
Be careful not to give the impression you're not
Have private jokes; allude to things said before
Carefully share secrets, but keep some mystery
Subtly let know you're easy to get *only* for them
Play it right and sweep them off their feet!
Encourage a little insecurity, no "heart on sleeve"
Be unpredictable, indifferent to opinion, casual.
Use silence, irregular attention, competition, break a date, understay welcome,
drop cold—temporarily
Be willing to walk out if necessary
Always at least appear to be one step behind
e.g. "Oh, I agree. I don't want to get serious either!"
"I enjoy talking with you, and just want to be friends"

But be careful of being so competitive *you* want someone just because *they* are a challenge!

 May end up with someone you really don't want

Be a knight in shining armor (if a guy)

 Fight the battles, treat with respect, sweep off feet

Be patient: people run from early commitment

 Take one step at a time, slowly, and stay one step behind

 Move ahead, then back up

Take time and effort to understand how

 And love them the way they want to be loved

Be a mystery, not an "open book". Simple people are boring

 Figure a way to create curiosity

 It should take a lifetime to understand each other

Use touch very carefully and very subtly—used right it can cause ignition!

Amicability

We grow dependent on those who supply emotional needs:

Friendship, attention, understanding, acceptance, affirmation, appreciation, affection, trust

Communicate: *Focus* on them, find *their* hot buttons, mirror, synchronize, compliment, use their vocabulary, talk of feelings and personal things, emphasize "we", *listen*

Discuss interests, values, and goals important to them

Identify and discuss complementary qualities

 Imply you are a team against the world

Identify and support their image of themselves. Give strokes

Get them doing little things for you

 [And do things for them, but *not* as quid pro quo]

Early on, encourage their independence, freedom, and noncommitment—remember, it is *friendship* that is needed

 Be sincere and willing to be somewhat vulnerable

Encourage them to open up by, *carefully*, opening up yourself.

 This is one of the risks of relationships

Never criticize or give unsolicited advice

 Listen, restate, and support

Be understanding/empathetic/sensitive

Have a sense of humor; return good for evil—bite your tongue!

 Don't get paranoid or make mountains out of molehills

 Be easy and fun to be with. Don't be defensive

 Be able to laugh together

Respect

Be worthy of admiration: Character, confidence, emphasize your similarities, have status, humor, flexibility, self control

 Respect must be earned: develop character, continue growth

Treating with respect not same as respecting

To great extent, people treat you as you expect and require

How you treat yourself is critical – figure you should know

You must be the kind of person you want to be with

You can't live a free and easy lifestyle and hope to attract a person of character

People are most attracted to independence, self-reliance, some aloofness (which women think is "confidence")

Radiate positive self-image, confidence, direction, growth

Act, don't react. Avoid defensiveness and "fishing"

Signs of low self esteem or insecurity in the relationship

Always have a plan—be decisive

Be attractive: Groom and dress carefully

But be sensitive and willing to compromise

Always look for the other's point of view

Accept defeat gracefully, when necessary

But don't allow yourself to be manipulated

Confront negative behavior diplomatically and empathetically, but firmly

Don't argue, but don't back down if right

Pick battles carefully

Always treat them with respect—affirm feelings even if disagree. You may agree to disagree

Expect, affirm, and assist their growth, on their terms

If you ever get caught checking out someone else, it is disrespectful. You deserve a swift kick!

Equity

Maybe not romantic or democratic, but a "bargaining" process

Must be convinced getting a "good deal"

Someone of *equal value*: Love is not blind

Cinderella had to have equities to balance lack of status

May be similar or offsetting mix of characteristics   If not similar, must at least balance, or violates nature

"Chips" include looks, money, status, knowledge, personality, manners, character, and inner nature

A cost-benefit analysis: What does each offer?

What is the perception you create? How can you improve?

Build equity: Lose weight, look sharp, learn, etc.

More even a marriage is, the better chance to succeed

If not similar, conflict is continual

One will begin to condescend, other to over-compensate

Equities may change after marriage, e.g. weight, money

Changes can destroy the relationship

CHARACTER TRAITS

People are a balance and blend of qualities and characteristics

It requires time, experience, and insight to identify them

In self as well as in partner

Must "know thyself" before can know another

Must have good relationship with self first

These characteristics relate to the areas of creating and sustaining a relationship, as discussed above

Some of these characteristics can be discovered quickly

Others take a long time to be certain

Even sanity can be faked

Consider potential partner for similar, complementary, conflicting traits

Use dating to identify the important characteristics

Then look for someone who has them

If not compatible, no point continuing a relationship

Similarity of characteristics builds unity

Differences cause conflict, negotiation, adaptation, compromise, capitulation, even separation

Healthy characteristics require continuous development

Self-responsibility and independence are prerequisite

Goal is interdependence

Must progress thru dependence and independence

Secure with own worth; don't always have to be right

One with self respect formulates opinions carefully, defends self fairly, *loves truth* more than winning, and lives with it even when unpleasant, is not arrogant, allows others their opinions

Authentic—not phony or role player; intimate and honest

Adaptable [by choice and habit]—helps resolve differences

Deadly characteristics will destroy a relationship

E.g. Dishonesty, jealousy, insecurity, sociopathy, extreme neuroticism, depression, uncontrolled anger, manic-depressive or obsessive-compulsive behavior, dependence

Sociopathy [tend to be likable and charming]: Phony, no conscience, dishonest, impulsive, disregard other's rights

As Lincoln said, "Can fool some people all the time"

Neurosis [all have some!]: Excessive guilt, shame, or anxiety

Inability to see and deal with problems realistically

Continue to do the same things, even tho they don't work

Continue to do things that do "work" even tho dysfunctional

[I've long said a neurotic is one who looks in the mirror and says, "What can I do today to really screw up your life!"]

Personality traits to analyze for compatibility:

Extravert/introvert

Intense/easygoing

Logical/intuitive

Humorous/serious
Strong/dependent
Judgmental/tolerant
Sophisticated/ingenuous and naive
Demonstrative/reserved
All these things blend into a unique personal "style"
      You either like and accept it, or you don't
    Need not necessarily be similar, but complementary
    Can you get on without frequent conflict and negotiation?
Characteristics that should be similar in a relationship:
    Physical attractiveness
    Conflict style: Volatile, validating, avoiding [see infra]
    Religion and spirituality
    Character
    Health and fitness
Sex drive
Social skills and status
Ambition
Income saved
Sense of responsibility
Lifestyle
Privacy required
Energy level
Amount of time desired together
How time together is used
Recreation
Politics
Hygiene
Area to live
House and decor
Issues to discuss and negotiate between partners (All associations, including marriage, are a continuing negotiation):
    Way love is shown and desired
    Expected roles and responsibilities
Power distribution
Conflict resolution
Children (hers, his, theirs)
Sources and use of income
Risk taking (physical, financial, etc.)
Inlaws
Friendships with opposite sex
Weight and fitness
Hobbies and interests

Handling sickness
Social involvement
Vacations
Leisure time activities

EVALUATION/COMPARISON OF TRAITS

Once someone is pushing the hot buttons, it's time to objectively evaluate the following "*SPISE*" characteristics

Both self and a potential partner

Even if this analysis does not sound "romantic"

It takes maturity and wisdom to consider these things fairly

Not necessarily the higher the score, but the closer the correlation the better the chance for success [Equity as well as things in common]. A few points can be a big difference.

Essentially, this analysis can tell you "no" but it can't tell you "go"

It can show conflicts, problem areas, and hidden "bombs"

(Rating: 10 = Top 1%, 9 = Top 10%, etc)

CHARACTERISTIC	RATING	
	Self	Partner
1-SPIRITUAL		
SERVICE		
RELIGION		
MORALITY		
ETHICS		
2-PHYSICAL		
AGE		
LOOKS		
FIGURE/BUILD		
FITNESS & HEALTH		
GROOMING & DRESS		
3-INTELLECTUAL		
INTELLIGENCE		
DEPTH		
KNOWLEDGE		
COMMON INTERESTS		
CONTINUAL LEARNING		
EARNING CAPACITY		
4-SOCIAL		
PERSONAL "STYLE"		
SOCIAL SKILLS		
SOPHISTICATION		
CONGENIALITY		
5-EMOTIONAL		

SANITY		
MATURITY		
LOYALTY		
CONFIDENCE		
TOUGHNESS		
AMBITION		
LACK OF NEEDINESS		
NON-CONTROLLING		
WORK ETHIC		
ENERGY		
ENTHUSIASM		
SENSE OF HUMOR		
ROMANTICISM		
LIBIDO		
NO GAME PLAYING		
SELF ESTEEM [CAST]: Conscience, Achievement, Service, No negative "Tapes"		

A RELATIONSHIP NEEDS "CLASS"

Once created, *sustaining* romantic love takes "CLASS"

   Developed on 3 levels: Physical, Emotional, Spiritual

C – Things in *Common*

Together: Read, learn, play, have a hobby, etc.

   Plan things to do together. Life is short, so do it

   List all the things you want to do. Check them off

   Work together in some way to serve others

But not just common likes and interests—least important

Also common goals, principles, attitudes, values, equities, and concept of and commitment and loyalty to the relationship—in mind as well as acts

Must have essentially similar conscious and subconscious ideas of what a relationship should be or it will not succeed

   Requires careful consideration, discussion, negotiation

L – *Like* each other

Like their "style": Cocky, introverted, loquacious, etc.

Like their habits and personal characteristics

Like the things that make them different and unique

Like just being together, comfortable talking—or not

   All the facets of companionship

Show by Scout motto: Do good turn (for each other) daily

   Do one thing special together each day [besides *that*!]

A – *Accept* each other—the really difficult one!

It is said men marry hoping she will never change; women marry hoping he will. Both are disappointed . . .

Everyone has characteristics their partner does not like
*These must be accepted, or the relationship broken off
Change is not likely, and must not be demanded
Mutual respect, and getting along, requires this
Tolerance and forgiveness are difficult but *imperative*
Might as well relax and appreciate what they are
If there is abuse, addictions, philandering, or dishonesty
Get out immediately!
Otherwise only have a right to quit when you have completely earned it, by
doing everything possible to make it work
Flexibility and adaptability are imperative to get along
It's often a matter of perspective, e.g. farm wife: "No, I
don't mind when my husband's boots bring in mud—they also bring in my
husband!"
Axiomatic: Must give to receive—*in each area*
No tradeoffs! e.g. supporting the family but avoiding verbal intimacy; fixing
dinner, but then having a headache . . . .
No *quid pro quo*: giving must be free. This is loving
Feel good for the giving—not dependent on the response
Growth of each partner is important
But its direction is the individual's *own* choice
S – Sex
The chemistry has to be there, for most people
Sex is the ultimate selfless/selfish act
There must be total loyalty, in thought as well as act
The better it is for the other, the better for you
For many, it's the thing that makes life worth living
Oprah claims if American women are lousy lovers it's because American men
are lousy lovers
True! For men, sex is almost a mechanical function
Any problem is almost always the man's fault
Unless she has a specific physical or emotional problem
This may require professional help
Usually he fails to be caring, patient, or skillful
For men, sexual response is easy
Women often must learn to respond
The man must teach them
S – Service
Giving service is requisite to love
Taking without giving is like the Dead Sea
Fair is fair! But not quid pro quo
COMMUNICATING

Women forever complain about the lack of—and they are right!

Without it the marriage fails, whether they stay together or not

Gottman found this common element in 2000 marriages

And that means real communication

With understanding, caring, and empathy

A man was deep in prayer. Suddenly God spoke to him. "I have searched your heart and determined it to be pure. Because you have been faithful to me in all ways, I will grant you one wish you ask for."

The man thought and said, "I have few needs, but I've always wanted to go to Hawaii. I'm deadly afraid of flying. Will you build a bridge across the sea?"

God laughed and said, "I could do it, but it would take a huge amount of your world's resources. Your request is very materialistic; a little disappointing."

The man thought about it for a long while. Finally, he said, "Here's the deal, Lord. My wife always says I don't care and I'm insensitive. So I wish I could understand women. I want to know how they feel inside and what they're thinking when they give me the silent treatment. I want to know why they're crying. I want to know what makes them happy. I want to know what they really mean when they say, 'Nothing'. So that's my wish, God: I just want to be able to understand them."

After a long silence God spoke: "You want two lanes on that bridge or four?"

Men and women do speak different languages

A real effort must be made, by both, to understand

Arguments result from not understanding the differences

A different vocabulary, e.g: love, respect, intimacy:

Women say, "You're not listening". It means you don't agree

To women, love is a feeling; to men it is how one acts

To men, respect is an attitude, to women it is how they

are treated—basically a reversal!

Everyone knows the different definitions for intimacy!

(From *Men Are From Mars*):

Women exaggerate and generalize

Men take them literally

Women talk for intimacy and validation

Men exchange info and facts

Women talk about feelings and people

Men about things and goals

Women complain to get sympathy and validation

Men perceive as an attack, or try to give solutions

Women talk to explore meaning

Men think first—which women perceive as indifference or trying to lie

Women show listening by asking questions

Men resent a multiplicity of detailed questions

Women apologize to show caring

Men when they are wrong
Women blame men to cause guilt so men will show caring
Men become angry because they take it personally
Women give advice whenever they see a "mistake"
Men want advice only if they ask for it
Both posture to conceal hurt, guilt, etc.
Developing listening skills
Focus on the other person, block out all else
Pay attention. . . and pay attentions
Allow them to finish what they are saying
Don't interrupt; be sure you understand the meaning
Listen carefully and actively; restate what they say
Avoid arguing; be sure you know what they mean
Not only understand, be sure they agree you understand
Be non-judgmental, by separating act from actor
Do not get angry; validate even if disagree
Strive to keep the volume down – even whisper
Developing verbal intimacy
Women demand; men avoid—don't know what's demanded
Not comfortable with the process because don't know how
Self-understanding, and willingness, are necessary
Mutual spiritual base is required [need not be religious]
Always speak truthfully, but tactfully
Share inner self: feelings, goals, fears
Describe feelings to create similar feelings in the other
Discuss: commitment, emotions, experiences, things in common, things diverse, personal characteristics
This intimacy will confirm oneness—or lack of it!
Potentially an enjoyable, unifying experience
Rationalization is the most practiced human skill
Men are probably more likely to be outright liars
But truth is often seen as relative (rationalized) by women
Women often seem to agree with the following excerpt from the novel *Madeleine*, written by a woman. (An attorney has been retained to defend Madeleine against a charge of murder. He is in the habit of going to his father for council. His father, for some time, has been resting in the local cemetery . . .):
He knelt at the base of the moonlit stone.
"Father", he whispered.
Yes, son?
"I am confused, father. I am sure she lied in her statement, and yet I trust her absolutely".
Oh, yes, indeed!

"Don't mock me, father. How can I believe that she is lying and trust her word absolutely at the same time?"

I do not mock you, son. Women cannot lie. To survive in society, men need to depend on truth. Women can survive only by saying what is needed, not what is true. For a woman, necessity is the equivalent of truth.

"Father, you are harsh".

I am not harsh. We become what we need to be.

"Father, should I believe her?"

No.

"Then I should disbelieve her?"

No.

"Oh father, what then?"

Trust her!

But you had better be sure your trust is justified!

Trust, by either partner, is not a feeling and not an attitude

It is something you should *choose* whether to do

The choice must be based on reality

Would you trust them with your money? [But *don't*]

Would you trust them with your deepest secret?

If a woman, would you trust him to give his life to save yours? That is a man's job, when circumstances require

If trust is violated, and *if* the problem is resolved, then trust must be *chosen* once again

INTUITION

"Les femmes, they like to think it is a special weapon that the good God has given them, and for every once it shows them the truth, at least nine times it leads them astray." - Hercules Poirot, famous fictional detective

Or, as Rupert Hughes said, "Women's intuition is the result of a million years of not thinking!"

[From *Intelligence Came First*, Smith, ed.]:

Right-brained intuition is imperative to the creative process

But intuition is only valuable if it is accurate

Otherwise it is counterproductive and destructive

Intuition is frequently misinterpreted when received

In mature adults, intuition develops through series of planes

10 to 14 years: emotion is seat of intuition [Marcault]

Logical thought is subservient. Many don't outgrow this

Later (13 to 18), it *should* pass from emotion to reason

Only then becomes effective tool in decisions

Reasoning must follow the flash of intuition

Intuition takes *hard work*, e.g. Einstein

Some are just too lazy to think

It takes no effort to "intuit"

Least mature likely to claim greatest intuition
Stuck on dumb!
Mature people refer to this as "rationalization"
Best to have balance of left and right brain hemispheres
If one side dominates, it better be the left
    God help you if you are right brain dominant!
Test own intuitive maturity by analyzing results
Reality is the fire in which intuition must be tried
Be careful in accepting anyone else's intuition
Particularly if intuition violates common sense
"Intuition" often passed off as "inspiration"
Attitude is if God said it, who can argue?

EMOTIONAL CYCLES

(from *Men Are From Mars*)
Men and women have different, often conflicting, cycles
    Failure to understand causes conflict and paranoia
Men have a cycle of increasing and decreasing intimacy
    Men draw away under stress, want to be ignored
    Women think drawing away is rejection
        They encroach and get burned
        Men cannot give support at such times
    Men draw away because need independence and space
        Spending too much time together damages cycle
        Women must avoid chasing or punishing
Women's cycle is rise and fall at 3-5 week intervals
    Some relatively stable, others violently extreme
    Depth of trough depends on emotional ill health
        And on amount of intimacy and trust in the relationship
    When down, women need communication—not space!
        Men must not 1] feel attacked or 2] offer solutions
            Non-judgmental listening is critical
            Don't take it personal—even tho it seems so
    Trough is place to heal; which may require years
        Women need to feel safe, validated going into trough
Hardest times when trough and drawing away correspond

CONFLICT DYNAMICS

[from *WHY MARRIAGES SUCCEED* by Gottman]
Based on empirical data from studies of 2000 marriages
    Found much conventional wisdom is wrong
[Gottman does not point it out, but this info is subject to the partners being
otherwise compatible and motivated to stay together. Seems to assume that is
so since they got married]
Disagreements are healthy

People who never fight are likely in an unhappy marriage
Conflict is not negative—it's how it is handled
Most important each feel good about the interaction
Less important the problem be resolved
*The Magic Ratio: 5 to 1
Most important determinant to success in marriage:
5 positive emotional feelings for every negative one
Negatives: *Necessary* to a healthy marriage
One thing they do is keep up passion! Emotions fire us up
There will be differences, and these must be dealt with
Couples without conflict likely to end in divorce
Positives: Show interest, affection, caring, appreciation,
concern, empathy, acceptance, joke, share joy
A balance thermostat kicks in to turn up the positives
Sometimes have to force these
*Successful marriages develop 1 of 3 styles
Depends how emotional the partners are, and example of parents
Closer partners' conflict styles match, more likely to succeed
Couples must go thru negotiation and develop a style
Validating Style: Listen, understand, accept when don't agree
The usual idea of what a marriage *should* be
Little hostility, much mutual respect, mutual persuasion
Do a lot of active listening, mutual supporting
Avoidant Style: Minimize conflict, make light of differences
Little attempt made to solve issues: "Agree to disagree"
Do not talk things out: Sweep conflicts under carpet
Focus on shared vision of a strong marriage
Bond so strong can overlook disagreement
Volatile Style: Very open about expressing negative feelings
See selves as equals, interrupt each other often
Lots of negatives, but lots of positives too [5 to 1]
A lot of passion in the marriage—love "making up"
[Not good to fight in front of kids]
Unsuccessful marriages are characterized by a downward spiral:
Criticism, then Contempt/Defensiveness, then Stonewalling
The cycle becomes more and more difficult to break
Contempt is the primary indicator of imminent failure
"Criticism" is general vs. "complaining" which is specific
Complaining is good, and easily handled if talk fairly
Complaints become criticism if they go unheeded
Contempt is the intention to insult and psychologically abuse
Attack sense of self, stop admiring, become abusive
Done by insults, name calling, sarcasm, mockery, body language

Defensiveness is the completely natural reaction to contempt and criticism
> But does not matter that you are right
>> It obstructs communication and nothing is resolved
> Must force self not to respond defensively
> Avoid by overlooking the attack
>> Look for the complaint behind it and respond to that
Stonewalling is *habitually* ignoring confrontation
> Partner becomes totally frustrated and begins to scream
> Stonewallers just trying to be neutral and avoid conflict
> Absolutely destructive; and 85% are men
If these 4 are not fixed the relationship is over
> Successful marriages invariably used repair mechanisms
>> These are not necessarily done in a conciliatory tone!
> Take "time-outs" when necessary
> Only respond to the complaint—ignore everything else
>> Agree in advance to stick to the complaint
> Express affection, even if forced
> Keep a sense of humor
> At times don't say anything, just listen
> Do not issue ultimatums or force issues
> Talk about *how* you are talking and arguing
> Men need to learn to embrace her anger, not sidestep it
>> Consciously look for resolutions
> Women need to learn to confront gently and calmly
>> Otherwise man will withdraw
> Both need to learn more acceptance
Fixing the problem is not the major issue, communicating is
Important thing is to remain calm, speak and listen non-defensively, validate each other, overlearn these principles so use them even when angry

CONFLICT RESOLUTION

Recognize that most disagreements aren't worth arguing about
> But people will go on and on . . . . They just want to be right
>> Argue for half an hour whether a color is blue or green
>> Never even listen to the other's point of view
> Listen to other couples – and recognize you may be similar
> At least 3 circumstances in which no chance to win an argument
>> Insanity, stupidity, and prejudice
2 types conflicts: 1] Those that tear down a relationship
2] Those that build it. Examine to see which is happening
Avoid pushing buttons everyone has—and spouse knows
> Avoid competing with each other, except if fun
> People pretty much treat you the way you require they do
>> If you are not treated right, it's your responsibility

Read and study *How To Win Friends and Influence People*
Follow the golden rule
Take responsibility: This is *my* problem—only I can solve it
Any other attitude means you can do nothing, have no power, are helpless:
"Blaming, complaining, and explaining"
>Counterproductive, even if true
>Actually *cause* the thing focused on—the thing feared
>Virtually *anything* can be fixed—if both *want* to!
>>Both must accept *full* responsibility
>Conflicts can be *good*, if handled well: bring together
Recognize there are many alternative ways to respond to conflict
>The instinctive way is probably the least effective
>Think of alternatives in advance, and plan the best response
>>E.g. use humor instead of becoming hurt and defensive
The basic questions: 1) Do you want to be married to each other 2) Are you willing to pay the price
If answer to both, by both, is "yes" recognize part of price is to communicate, negotiate, compromise, resolve
>It's no good trying to be in a relationship alone [D.J.]
Write down what each expects from all areas of marriage
Discuss, negotiate, reach agreement—a contract
Destructive conflict comes from selfish focus
>Causes denial, withdrawal, explosion, manipulation
>Competition is great—but not in marriage!
>Agree each has veto power in mutual decisions
>>*No one made either boss! Learn leadership
Attempts to control are a leading cause of conflicts
>Most conflicts relate to attempts to control
>Managers attempt to control, leaders to influence
>>Influence requires truth, persuasion, patience, love
>If control necessary because spouse anti-social then get out
>Otherwise control is *always* the result of low self esteem
>>Most bad behavior is the result of insecurity, not evil intent
>>"If they are nice even when I'm mean they must love me"
>>"If they do what I want, even when unfair, must love me"
>>"If they do what I want, I must be right"
>>Recognize it, and exercise self-discipline to stop
>People with good self esteem do not need to control others
>>Recognize ultimately all we can control is ourselves
>>>And they're fine with that! No one made anyone boss
>>>Way to control self is by controlling thoughts
Arguments kill love, but so will suppression of a problem
Often occur, even when trying, because one responds as wants to be

responded to, not as other wants
> Woman feels invalidated, and will not listen to "reason"
>> Man focuses on being right, instead of caring
> Very likely to occur when emotional cycles are at odds
>> At such times, woman should talk to friends
>> Removing pressure helps man out of withdrawal

4 bad stances in argument: Men tend to fight or withdraw
> Women tend to fake agreement or give in
>> May be depressed and not know why
>> Giving in when right shows a lack of self respect

Refusal to give in when wrong shows dishonesty, stupidity, or low self esteem. Care to pick one?

To resolve a conflict, do the following

Recognize you love each other, and will get through it

Exercise self control, no matter how difficult
> Even if can't control how feel can control words and acts

Have no right to damage another's self esteem—especially one's mate
> If you have to, chew off your tongue!

Describe problem, in simple, not loaded, *facts*

Express *feeling*: "I feel. . ." Avoid "you". Keep it light

Specify what you *want*—don't make them guess

Identify *consequences*: Preferably good thing will happen
> Decide in advance a positive consequence to offer
>> Negative consequence only if positive doesn't work

Women cause conflicts by unsolicited advice and by failure to be direct
> When questioning, tone of voice indicates judgment
> Rhetorical questions aggravate men!

Much of being upset relates to old issues
> The upset person may not even realize it
>> Overreacts and resents when pointed out
> A little bump does not hurt—except in an old wound
> If a man's past is brought up, he withdraws
>> If woman's, her self esteem crashes

Constructive conflict is based on responsibility, respect, and unequivocal commitment to the relationship
> Each must be *absolutely sure* of the other's commitment
> Each must agree the other has a right to feel as does
> Avoid defensiveness and fight down paranoia
>> Most people meet anger with anger—Don't!

Choose fights carefully—most things are just not worth fighting about
> Keep a soft sense of humor
> Type A people really have to struggle with this

Try to understand each other fully re the problem
    Most arguments, neither understands other's point
    Not listening while other talks: Planning own argument
    Instead of arguing, ask, "Why do you believe that?"
Find *something* to agree about
    Emphasize areas of agreement
Specify points of disagreement [write if it helps]
    Leads to discussion, not disagreement and conflict
You can't argue with stupidity, don't even try
    When there is no interest in facts or logic
    Only way is with objective third party
Keep a sense of humor! Don't sweat the small stuff
    (It's all small stuff!) Try to laugh *together*
Relax, and quit trying so hard
Define and examine alternatives, and work out a resolution
Ignore extraneous issues which just increase conflict
    Get to core of problem to find solution
Celebrate agreement! Reinforce positive behavior
    It will then tend to keep happening—everybody wins!
Work for win/win. A lot of talk about it these days
    Much is just lip service
    Takes great creativity if both *really* win
Finally: Forgiving is not a burden, it is an *opportunity*
To learn and demonstrate love and understand the atonement
    Just how big—or small—a person are you?
Many conflicts are the result of simply not knowing what to do or how to do it—there is no bad motive involved
    Need to recognize this and develop better responses
    The other needs to exercise tolerance and leadership
When really need to pour oil on troubled water
    Sincerely say: "I really miss it when we're not close"
    Learn to say with feeling, even when angry, "I love you"
    It will melt an iceburg!

PITCHING FITS AND OTHER BIZARRE BEHAVIOR

There are many kinds of irrational reactions to the inevitable conflicts in marriage, e.g. silent treatment, walking out, pitching fits, etc. Pitching fits is discussed as an example because it is one I have specifically experienced and studied. To deal effectively with this issue, two things must be recognized: 1] The fits are not their fault. In the past, someone very close—generally their parents—has caused deep injuries, and these injuries are the root of deep insecurities. The fits are the inappropriate symptom of terrible emotional pressures and an unconscious need to prove to themselves they are worthy of, and are receiving, love—a subconscious feeling that "if he puts up with this he must *really* love me". 2] A rational approach to dealing with such irrational behavior is not only ineffective, it is counterproductive. The only thing that can heal these injuries is unequivocal love and security. The husband is typically the only one who can provide this love, security, and healing. Smalley says a woman's emotional health is totally the husband's responsibility after five years of marriage.

Emotionally, women seem not like the sun, but more like the moon: they reflect the nature and quality of emotional light that comes from the man. Whether he likes it or not, the man is the emotional leader. Recognize this is controversial, but even staunch feminists seem this way (no doubt a cause for extreme anger and frustration!). For example, if the man is in a bad mood, she typically blames him; if the woman is in a bad mood, she blames him! If a woman has deep injuries, it is the husband's responsibility to help her heal, which can only occur during the fits. He does this by not taking her accusations personally, by affirming—though not necessarily agreeing with—her feelings (say, "I'm sorry you feel that way"), by giving love despite the fit, and, especially, by providing unquestioned security. Withdrawing or condemning—as a "rational" refusal to affirm extremely irresponsible behavior—is absolutely wrong, though it seems the reasonable thing to do. It feeds the insecurity and opens the wound. The husband must walk a fine line between capitulation and repudiation.

Women do not understand the reason for their feelings [Hormones, right!], and so they accuse the man of all kinds of bizarre things. But failure to provide unequivocal support during the fits is the failure about which they have a real right to complain, as it strikes at their deepest primal instinct. [Admittedly, in these women, this instinct is highly oversensitive. In some it can be a bottomless pit] Partly because of the nature of men, providing active love and support at such a time is difficult, but it is the only way a woman can be healed. In time, as she heals, the fits become fewer and less explosive.

FAITH IN RELATIONSHIPS
"Through faith, all things are possible"
This is nearly literally true, tho not quite the intended meaning. It really means that all things possible to be done are done thru faith. All success in *all* things is determined by faith: temporal as well as spiritual, in time and eternity
Faith does not have power to abrogate agency .
    Any attempt to do so is *wrong!*
    Attempts to control are always the result of low self esteem
    Attitude of "If they will put up with it, must really love me!"
Like other things, times in relationship when just want to quit
    Pressure builds to point feel like will explode
    Even tho know have no right to quit the relationship
        (Except abuse, drug addiction, dishonesty, or philandering)
    But thru faith, *any* two people can be happily married

Provided they are physically attracted, have a sound spiritual base, and *both* exercise faith

All problems can be overcome if both *will*

    Faith of one cannot overcome free agency of other

    Divorce inevitable only if partners won't exercise faith

Faith is not one principle, but three

    1] Belief, 2] Action, 3] Power – each leads to the next

Faith is a literal power. If one believes, in faith, and acts, in faith, God will provide the power, thru faith.

    Even—or especially—if it seems impossible

    Faith has power to do the impossible

    Faith gauged by how much impossible is accomplished

Acting in faith is far more important than believing: refuse to quit!

Seek for guidance, strength, and commitment thru prayer

Faith must be exercised according to true principles

    It requires complete honesty

    Do what is right, let the consequence follow

    Trust the Lord at all times and in all things

        Even when don't work out as desired, *trust him!*

        Do best you are able to, so *can* trust him

    It requires the exercise of absolute *will* and control of

    thoughts. Faith is, to a great extent, a *choice*

Negative, defeatist, grass-is-greener thoughts must be quelled

Focus on the positive

    Think of every way to make the relationship work

    It requires an attitude of "I will never, *never* quit!"

There must be an absolute commitment (subject to a similar commitment by one's partner)

        You can't keep a back door open

But refusing to quit is not enough. A process of faith required:

    Have to keep struggling upward, not just hang by fingertips

    Desire-Decision-Plan-Commitment-Action—Power

    Requires doing *everything* that is reasonably possible

        No attitude of "I'll stay, if you fix it!"

No attitude of "I'm miserable, but do it because I must"

    "*I* am responsible" (subject to *your* being willing)

    Living by faith is doing the best with what you've got

Remember: After the trial come the blessings

    Even if, in rare cases, divorce is inevitable

    Trials and pain are a necessary and proper part of life

        Bad things do happen to good people—for a purpose

        All experiences are intended to develop faith

        Use them for that purpose—be grateful!

To strengthen faith, always remember the eternal goal
    Think about what will matter 100 years from now

PARENTING

The most important job we have – with the least training
    Only "training" for most people is their own parents
        For good, bad, or indifferent
    The world and society make parenting a really tough job
        Dishonesty, immorality, drugs, conflicts, etc, etc
        Pillory Clinton said, "It takes a village"
            Or, as the communists said it, "It takes the State"
            That is *wrong*. What it takes is a good family
            That is the way God ordained it
            A village can be an adjunct, but a damn poor substitute
Kids need, and are entitled to, certain basic needs:
    Love, safety, shelter, food, security, training, discipline
    Failure to provide these needs is criminal
    Same as with spouse, need to discover how kids want love
Parents do not, however, have to be perfect
    If God required that, he would have them raised by angels
    But need to do the best possible, including learning how
    One day kids will be adults – and remember things you did
        Those memories can be very happy, or embarrassing!
Many kids grow up out of control from a very young age
    A real pain to their parents and others around them
No right to hurt others, disrespect others, especially adults, or interfere with others doing things they have a right to do
    It is the nature of children to push the limits from very early
        The stronger their will, the stronger they push
            Too often, the child's will is the stronger!
            Keeps at it till the parent is ground down
        To discipline a child requires a stronger will than the child
            That does not mean *force*, it means *will*
    Kids learn to do what works – parents *teach* them
    Worst thing is to teach them instant gratification
            Learn to get what want by unsocial methods, eg. Whining
            Keep at it, inexorably, till the parent is ground down
            Play on parents' guilt till they give in
                Children learn opposite of what needed to work in life
Many rebel sometime during their teens
    Cause generally related to one of three things, or all:
Parents are too lazy or indifferent to take responsibility
Parents are over-controlling, critical, or abusive
Parents can't deal with a strong-willed kid

Children actually want, as well as need, boundaries
  A child without boundaries, paradoxically, is not happy
    Make themselves miserable, as well as others
  But those boundaries must be reasonable, fair, consistent
"Reproving betimes with sharpness, but then showing love"
    The child must be given all latitude possible
      Otherwise they can never learn self-responsibility
      And they will rebel continually as they grow
The child must learn that fair, reasonable boundaries absolutely *cannot* be crossed without serious consequences
  Both parents must consistently commit, together
  If "time outs" or persuasion will do it, fine [Good luck!]
    If not, then more is required, but it *must* be done
      Every kid different, and requires a different approach
  One of best ways is to count to 3
    With consistency, child learns not to let you get to 3!
    No spanking, but a swat on the bottom is sufficient
    Send to room, alone. Allowed out when will behave
      No X-Box while there
Like the baby elephant tied to a stake: Learns he can't pull it out; and even when older still "can't"
From pre-speech times children need to:
Be taught what is right
Be encouraged and allowed to make as many decisions for themselves as they are capable and responsible
Be supported in their right to make all decisions possible.
Parents should take responsibility to teach, and to defend why a child isn't allowed to do something – not the other way around. No "Because I said so, and I'm the parent!"
  This must not be allowed to become interminable
    Explain valid reasons once, and that is the end
Be "allowed" to experience the consequences of their decisions, within maximum limits of safety
  J. Smith: "I teach correct principles and they govern selves"
Edmund Burke, 1796: "Men have a right to be free in direct proportion to their willingness to accept responsibility. Controls must be placed on the individual, and those controls must come from within or without."
  These principles are true of children as well as adults
    But forcing people is Satan's plan from the beginning
If training does not start very early, it becomes very difficult
  Cannot suddenly decide to allow a kid to make decisions
    And be responsible and accountable for them
  If try to change after child is trained wrong, he will pitch fits

Have to really commit to retraining or will get ground down
Have to force self to be firm and absolutely consistent

If training and discipline done correctly, children:
Do not rebel, because there is nothing to rebel against!
Learn to accept responsibility for themselves, because they are accountable
Develop attitudes and self discipline necessary for   happiness and success
resulting from good decisions

INSIGHTS

At various times, I have had insights into relationships that have changed—
sometimes shattered—my perspective. These have come from experience,
reading, thought, and the counsel of others. (It seems, however, as if the
insight often comes too late for the current problem. Hopefully, insights will
come in time for you.)

Relationships, and particularly with one's spouse, are the single possession in
life that can continue to provide satisfaction after being obtained. They are
worth it! Learn and follow the principles, and then relax and enjoy it!

Everything in a relationship is *my* responsibility. If I do not accept this as a
reality I am helpless; there is nothing I can do when there is a problem.

Men and women's emotions are ruled by primal instincts. Marriage cannot be
expected to be a union of two rational, independent people. Primal needs are
too powerful, and must be met for the relationship to succeed. How neurotic
the need is depends on the emotional health of the person.

A woman wants—and is entitled to—a knight in shining armor, in the sense of
meeting her primal instincts and romantic needs. It's his job to support her, to
slay the dragons (and the spiders, and everything in between), and to put her
on a little bit of a pedestal.

People have to be loved the way they want to be loved, or they will not even
realize they are being loved.

Conflicts are, of course, inevitable. The important thing is that they can spiral
up in a vortex of healing and a closer relationship or down in a whirlpool of
destruction.

Everyone has a personal emotional "style" that determines how they relate,
including arguing. Differences in style can destroy the relationship, especially
if one is volatile and one an avoider.

In relationships and in all associations, there is too much management in this
world, and not enough leadership. The latter is difficult. But no one was
appointed boss!

When there are two sides to the story, at least one is probably a lie.

Women seem to be like the moon, not the sun. Like it or not, their emotions
inevitably reflect the man and are *his* responsibility. That does not make him
boss either.

Women with an extreme need for security pitch fits. [I suppose some men also
do this.] At such times, even their virtues can become vices. The rational

response is to refuse to participate, as an effort to discourage them, but love, affirmation, and unquestioned security are the only way to offer healing. *Everyone* is insecure in some ways (and knowing this can be a weapon for self defense or a tool to help others). Many women and men fake confidence and security. To the extent they do so, there is a violent need for continuous expressions of unconditional security. Running on ego is like a tire with a hole in it: it's got to be pumped up continually. If you chose a mate like that then— like it or not—you got the job of pumping.

Many times people respond to things others say and do in defensive, dysfunctional ways simply because they have not learned a better way. How you feel is largely involuntary, how you respond is a *choice*.

"Playing small does not serve the world. There is nothing enlightened about shrinking so that others won't feel insecure around you. We were made to manifest the glory of God", according to Nelson Mandela. And as Eleanor Roosevelt said, "No one can make you feel inferior without your permission". Small-minded, insecure people are deeply offended by small, unintentional slights; big people handle affronts with relative equanimity. But their self-respect may cause them to leave.

*THE 10 KEYS TO A SUCCESSFUL RELATIONSHIP

The inner struggle:

♥Strive to live the Gospel: "Do unto the other as you would have them do unto you", "Cleave unto thy spouse and none else", "Have joy with thy spouse"

♥Control your thoughts: Every negative or sinful thought is a chip in the foundation of your faith

♥Do the "SPISE" evaluation, yourself and together: Spiritual, Physical, Intellectual, Social, Emotional

♥Build self esteem [not ego!] "CAST": Conscience, achievement, service, no negative "tapes"

The struggle together:

♥*Creating* a relationship requires "CARE": C: Chemistry, A: Amicability [friendship], R: Respect, E: Equity

♥*Sustaining* a relationship, once created, also takes "CLASS": C: Things in common, L: Like each other, A: Acceptance, S: Sanity, S: Sexual compatibility

♥Discover the Five Love Languages together: Verbal, Quality time, Gifts, Service, Touch

♥Maintain the Magic Ratio: 5 compliments for every complaint

♥Develop a common conflict style: Validating, Avoidant, Volatile

♥Faith, as in all things, is imperative. Develop the relationship through its *three* principles: Belief, Action, Power

INANUTSHELL

Of all the principles for a good relationship discussed above, a few [marked in the text by "*"] stand out as determinative:

*Relationships are the one thing we can obtain in life that can provide increasing satisfaction. Their value is inestimable.

*Keep trying to have fun, and never, *never* give up!

*Love is a decision and a commitment. Two questions: Do you really want a relationship? Are you willing to pay the price?

*Nobody made either partner boss.

*Neither partner has a right to demand change in the other. It won't happen by force!

*Work on the 10 Keys, listed above, separately and together.

*The bottom line: Are you building the kind of relationship where you want to be with them more than anything else in this world. Does your partner want to be with you more than anything else in this world? It's a two-way street to the greatest happiness.

Finally, from *ALL'S WELL THAT ENDS WELL*, by William Shakespeare:

"Tell me the reason why thou wilt marry."
"My poor body requires it, I am driven by the flesh!"
"Is this all your reason?"
"I have other, holy reasons: I have been a wicked creature
        and do marry that I may repent."
"Thy marriage, sooner than thy wickedness!"

Hopefully, this outline will help you repudiate the prediction.